Download the Gunner Goggles App Now!

Go to the App Store from your iPhone or iPad and search for **Gunner Goggles**

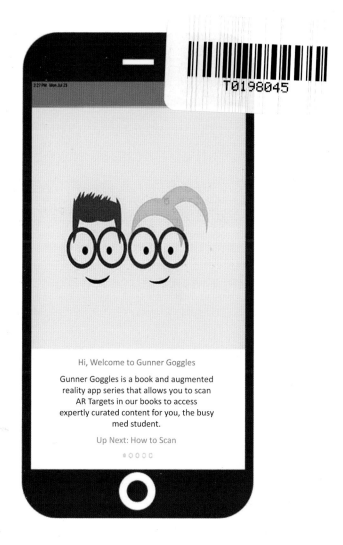

Each Gunner Goggles specialty has its own app; you can purchase other titles at:
ElsevierHealth.com/GunnerGoggles

GUNNER GOGGLES

Family Medicine

HONORS SHELF REVIEW

EDITORS:

Hao-Hua Wu, MD
Resident, Department of
Orthopaedic Surgery
University of California–San
Francisco
San Francisco, California

Leo Wang, MS, PhD
Perelman School of Medicine
University of Pennsylvania
Philadelphia, Pennsylvania

FACULTY EDITORS:

Katherine Margo, MD
Associate Professor of Family
Medicine and Community Health
Hospital of the University of
Pennsylvania
Philadelphia, Pennsylvania

Judy Chertok, MD
Clinical Assistant Professor of Family
Medicine and Community Health
Hospital of the University of
Pennsylvania
Philadelphia, Pennsylvania

ELSEVIER

ELSEVIER

1600 John F. Kennedy Blvd.
Ste 1800
Philadelphia, PA 19103-2899

GUNNER GOGGLES FAMILY MEDICINE, HONORS SHELF REVIEW   ISBN: 978-0-323-51034-9

Notices

Knowledge and best practice in this field are constantly changing. As new research and experience broaden our understanding, changes in research methods, professional practices, or medical treatment may become necessary.

Practitioners and researchers must always rely on their own experience and knowledge in evaluating and using any information, methods, compounds, or experiments described herein. In using such information or methods they should be mindful of their own safety and the safety of others, including parties for whom they have a professional responsibility.

With respect to any drug or pharmaceutical products identified, readers are advised to check the most current information provided (i) on procedures featured or (ii) by the manufacturer of each product to be administered, to verify the recommended dose or formula, the method and duration of administration, and contraindications. It is the responsibility of practitioners, relying on their own experience and knowledge of their patients, to make diagnoses, to determine dosages and the best treatment for each individual patient, and to take all appropriate safety precautions.

To the fullest extent of the law, neither the Publisher nor the authors, contributors, or editors, assume any liability for any injury and/or damage to persons or property as a matter of products liability, negligence or otherwise, or from any use or operation of any methods, products, instructions, or ideas contained in the material herein.

Library of Congress Cataloging-in-Publication Data
Names: Wu, Hao-Hua, editor. | Wang, Leo, editor. | Margo, Katherine,
    editor. | Chertok, Judy, editor. | Barkley, Kaitlyn, MD, editor.
Title: Gunner goggles family medicine : honors shelf review / editors,
    Hao-Hua Wu, Leo Wang ; faculty editors, Katherine Margo, Judy
    Chertok ; question editor, Kaitlyn Barkley.
Description: Philadelphia : Elsevier, [2019] | Includes bibliographical
    references.
Identifiers: LCCN 2017051047 | ISBN 9780323510349 (pbk. : alk. paper)
Subjects: | MESH: Family Practice | Test Taking Skills | User-Computer
    Interface | Study Guide
Classification: LCC R834.5 | NLM WB 18.2 | DDC 610--dc23 LC record
available at https://lccn.loc.gov/2017051047

Executive Content Strategist: Jim Merritt
Senior Content Development Specialist: Dee Simpson
Publishing Services Manager: Patricia Tannian
Senior Project Manager: Cindy Thoms
Senior Book Designer: Maggie Reid

Working together
to grow libraries in
developing countries

www.elsevier.com • www.bookaid.org

Printed in China

Last digit is the print number: 9   8   7   6   5   4   3   2   1

Gunner Goggles Honors Shelf Review Series

Gunner Goggles Family Medicine   978-0-323-51034-9

Gunner Goggles Medicine   978-0-323-51035-6

Gunner Goggles Neurology   978-0-323-51036-3

Gunner Goggles Obstetrics and Gynecology   978-0-323-51037-0

Gunner Goggles Pediatrics   978-0-323-51038-7

Gunner Goggles Psychiatry   978-0-323-51039-4

Gunner Goggles Surgery   978-0-323-51040-0

Contributors

QUESTION EDITOR

Kaitlyn Barkley, MD
Resident Physician
Department of Neurosurgery
University of Florida
Gainesville, Florida

CONTRIBUTING AUTHORS

Sila Bal, MD, MPH
Resident Physician
Massachusetts Eye and Ear
Boston, Massachusetts
Diseases of the Blood and Blood-Forming Organs

Isabella Bellon, MD
Resident Physician
Department of Family Medicine
University of Pennsylvania
Philadelphia, Pennsylvania
Mental Disorders

Lauren Briskie, MD
Resident Physician
Emergency Medicine
Christiana Care Health System
Newark, Delaware
Diseases of the Respiratory System

Jacob Charny, MD
Resident Physician
Department of Dermatology
University of Illinois College of Medicine
Chicago, Illinois
Disorders of the Skin and Subcutaneous Tissues

Jacob Cox, MD
Resident Physician
Department of Ophthalmology
Harvard Medical School
Boston, Massachusetts
Diseases of the Nervous System and Special Senses

Pujan Dave, MD
Resident Physician
Department of Ophthalmology
Johns Hopkins University
Baltimore, Maryland
Nutritional and Digestive Disorders

Jacques Greenberg, MD
Resident Physician
Department of Surgery
Cornell University
New York, New York
Renal, Urinary, and Male Reproductive System

Chevonne Parris-Skeete, MPH
Drexel University College of Medicine
Philadelphia, Pennsylvania
Endocrine and Metabolic Disorders

William Plum, MD
Resident Physician
Department of Ophthalmology
Columbia University
New York, New York
Diseases of the Respiratory System

Angela Ester Ugorets, MD
Resident Physician
Emergency Medicine
Cooper University
Camden, New Jersey
Disorders of the Skin and Subcutaneous Tissues

Junqian Zhang, MD
Resident Physician
Department of Dermatology
University of Pennsylvania
Philadelphia, Pennsylvania
Cardiovascular Disorders

Acknowledgments

"If I have seen further than others, it is by standing upon the shoulders of giants."

– Isaac Newton

We would like to thank the many exceptional innovators who helped transform our vision of *Gunner Goggles Family Medicine* into reality.

To our editorial team at Elsevier, thank you for your unrelenting support throughout the publication process. Jim Merritt believed in *Gunner Goggles* from day one and used his experience as an executive content strategist to point us in the right direction with respect to book proposal, product pitch, and manuscript development. Dee Simpson and Lucia Gunzel expertly guided us through manuscript submission and revision, no easy feat with two first-time authors. Maggie Reid collaborated with us closely to create the layout design and color schemes. Cindy Thoms and the copy editing team made sure our written content adhered to a high professional standard.

To the editors, authors, and student reviewers of *Gunner Goggles Family Medicine*, thank you for your scholarship and unwavering enthusiasm. Dr. Katherine Margo and Dr. Chertok took time out of their busy academic schedule to meticulously edit each chapter, and both provided numerous invaluable insights on how we could improve quality and accuracy. A number of outstanding residents and medical students contributed to the content of this textbook and provided us feedback on high-yield topics for the NBME Clinical Neurology Subject Exam, notably Dr. Sila Bal, Dr. Isabella Bellon, Dr. Lauren Briskie, Dr. Jacob Charny, Dr. Jacob Cox, Dr. Pujan Dave, Dr. Jacques Greenberg, Chevonne Parris-Skeete, Dr. William Plum, and Dr. Junqian Zhang.

To our augmented reality (AR) team, thank you for your creativity and dedication during the development of the *Gunner Goggles* AR application. Nadir Bilici, Brian Mayo, Vlad Obsekov, Clare Teng, and Yinka Orafidiya helped us develop and test the initial *Gunner Goggles* AR prototype. Tammy Bui designed the *Gunner Goggles* logo and AR app icon.

We would also like to thank the Wharton Innovation Fund for awarding us seed money to help pursue development of *Gunner Goggles* AR.

You all continue to inspire us, and we are incredibly grateful and deeply appreciative for your support.

-Hao-Hua and Leo

Contents

Introduction

Hao-Hua Wu, Leo Wang, and Katherine Margo

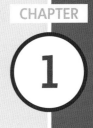

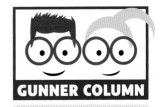

CHAPTER

1

I. The Gunner's Guide to a Better Test Score

Curious as to why certain classmates perform well on every exam? Frustrated by how few of these "gunner" peers share study secrets?

At *Gunner Goggles*, our goal is to reveal and demystify. By integrating *augmented reality (AR)* into this review book, we **reveal** how the best students approach topics, conceptualize complex disease and allocate study time efficiently. By organizing each topic according to the National Board of Medical Examiners (NBME) format, we **demystify** exam content and the types of questions one can expect on test day.

Of the tests medical students strive to conquer, shelf exams boast the highest ratio of importance to study resource quality. For instance, performance on shelf exams typically informs final clerkship grades, which are the most important criteria on the medical school transcript for residency application. Yet, there is no single authoritative study resource for the shelf across all disciplines. Most importantly, no current book specifically targets shelf exam prep. So students must rely on miscellaneous resources and anecdotal advice to get the job done.

In light of this void in authoritative test prep, we have created the *Gunner Goggles* series to provide you with the most effective shelf exam testing resource. *GG* stands out for three important reasons:

First, readers have the opportunity to enhance understanding of important shelf topics by utilizing the **AR** features on each page. With an iPhone or iPad, users can download the *Gunner Goggles* AR iOS app and use it to turn book figures into three-dimensional (3D) images, access high-yield videos and view pertinent digital media. More on how AR technology works can be found on page 2.

Second, *Gunner Goggles* provides a plethora of tips on how to manage time efficiently when studying for the shelf. Mnemonics and strategies for how to approach difficult

GUNNER COLUMN

concepts can be found in the blue "Gunner Column" to the right of each page. We also tell you how to *think* about these concepts so that Family Medicine never feels like a laundry list of items you simply have to memorize.

Third, this review book is written and organized optimally for shelf exam test prep. Each chapter is organized according to the NBME Clinical Science Subject Examination and USMLE Course Content outlines. In addition, a concise summary of how topics are tested prefaces each chapter.

As experts on the shelf exam, we understand how difficult it is to carve out time to study while juggling clinical responsibilities during your clerkship rotation. We also know that each student's learning curve is different based on timing of the rotation (first block vs. last block), year in medical school (MS3 vs. MD/PhD returning after graduate school), and future career interests (e.g., an aspiring orthopedic surgeon learning about obstetrics and gynecology). However, we believe that any student can perform well on the shelf with the right strategy and study resources.

We created this book anticipating the needs of all types of students, and hope that *Gunner Goggles* will be the most comprehensive, authoritative shelf exam review book that you ever use. We are confident that *Gunner Goggles* will enable you to achieve your test performance goals and stick it to your "gunner" classmates, whose advice, or lack thereof, you won't be needing after all.

II. Augmented Reality: A New Paradigm for Shelf Exam Test Prep

Think of AR as your best friend.

To use it, download the free *Gunner Goggles Family Medicine* application on your iPad or iPhone and create your own optional profile. Now with the application open, point your smart mobile camera at this page.

Notice how on your camera, there are now links you can click on, 3D figures you can rotate, and a video you can watch. You have just unlocked the AR features for this page!

Take a moment to play around with these AR features on your smart mobile device. The way this works is anytime you see the *Gunner Goggles* icon **gg** in the blue Gunner Column to the right or left, there is an AR feature accompanying the text with which you have the opportunity to interact with.

Still not convinced? Here are three reasons why AR is your ideal study companion.

gg AR

Introduction Video

gg AR

Contact

Presentation

AR breaks the boundaries of how information can be presented in this textbook.

Traditionally, if you wanted to learn about a disease in a review book, you would be expected to read and memorize a block of text similar to the following:

"Huntington disease (HD) is a GABAergic neurodegenerative disorder that is caused by an autosomal dominant mutation leading to CAG repeats on chromosome 4. Patients typically present in the fourth and fifth decade of life with chorea, memory loss, caudate atrophy on neuroimaging and motor impairment, depending on the variant. Although there is no cure for Huntington, the movement disorders associated with the disease, such as chorea, can be treated with drugs like tetrabenazine and reserpine to decrease dopamine release."

Having read (or most likely glazed) through that last paragraph, do you feel comfortable enough to answer questions about the genetics, presentation and treatment of Huntington right now? A week from now? Three weeks from now when you have to take your shelf exam?

Here's where AR comes in. Use your *Gunner Goggles* app to check out how we're able to present HD in different, memorable ways.

For visual learners, here's a video of an effective HD mnemonic →

99 AR
Huntington Disease Mnemonic

If you are an audio learner, here's a link to key points about Huntington for the shelf →

99 AR
Huntington Podcast

Forgot your neuroanatomy? Here's where the caudate is →

What's the difference between chorea, athetosis, and ballismus again? Chorea looks like this →

99 AR
The caudate nucleus is part of the basal ganglia

Now write a one-line description of Huntington in your own words in the margins of this page for future reference. It's much easier with AR right? Like we said, your best friend.

99 AR
Chorea patient example

Evaluation

The GG Family Medicine app has the potential to exponentially enhance how you can evaluate your own understanding of the material. Although not available with the first edition, we are in the process of developing a personalized question bank as well as a flashcards feature. Our vision is to allow you to scan a topic on the page for immediate access to relevant practice questions and flashcards. In future versions, you will also be able to create your own flashcard deck and track your mastery.

In addition the GG app can keep track of the AR Targets scanned and the Learning links viewed. These links are saved to a Link Library which you can view at any time. You can also like or dislike a Learning Link with an opportunity to provide us feedback for better resources available.

As development of the GG Family Medicine app is an ongoing process, we encourage and welcome your feedback. If you like the idea of having a personalized question bank and flashcard feature or have an idea for how we can improve the GG app to better serve your studying needs, please provide us feedback through an in-app message. You can also email us at GunnerGoggles@gmail.com.

Community Engagement

Studying for the shelf can be isolating. Our vision is to develop a feature in the GG Family Medicine that would allow you to connect with chapter authors and fellow readers. We are in the process of developing a medium in which shelf-related inquiries can be discussed among authors and readers through an optional short message system (SMS) feature.

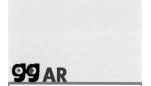

Given that the community engagement feature is in development and unavailable for the first edition, we welcome your input on how we can connect you with the people who will enable your test day success.

To provide feedback, please scan the page and vote. You can also email us GunnerGoggles@gmail.com for any comments or suggestions.

Augmented Reality Frequently Asked Questions

"Since augmented reality is integrated into *Gunner Goggle Family Medicine*, does this mean I have to pull out my iPad or iPhone for every page of the book?"

No, only if you need it. Some may use AR more than others depending on background and level of comfort with family medicine. For instance, you may already have a solid understanding of Huntington and only need to read the text as a refresher. On the other hand, if you are less comfortable with Huntington, the AR features are there just in case.

"Can't I just look up everything I don't know on my own? Why do I have to use the *Gunner Goggles* app?"

You can absolutely look things up on your own. But that takes time. And sometimes, you can't find the best reference or mnemonic. Our team of experts has already gone through the trouble of identifying potential sources of confusion for you and found the perfect resources. In the *Gunner Goggles* app, we have compiled the slickest and most concise resources one can use to better understand a topic. Videos, audio files, and images are first vetted by subject experts for accuracy of content. They are then evaluated by students like yourself for utility of content to enhance test performance. Only resources with the most Gunner votes are embedded into each page.

"What if a link doesn't work or I want something on the page to change?"

Please tell us! Another advantage of AR is that we can immediately receive and implement your feedback. Just use the *Gunner Goggles* app to text us your concerns and our tech support team will respond ASAP!

III. Study Smart: Mnemonics and Gunner Study Tips

Even with incredible AR features at your disposal, you won't be able to optimize exam performance unless you know how to study. Below are the four most important things one can do to study for the Family Medicine shelf under the time restraints imposed by clerkships.

Understand the Organizing Principle

The easiest way to save time and perform well on the shelf is to understand how a specific disease or concept fits into the big picture. For instance, knowing the buzz words, diagnostic steps and treatment plan for ulcerative colitis will likely lead to only one correct answer on the test. However, understanding that UC is a disease of hindgut and midgut, and knowing how to differentiate GI disorders based on location in the gut can help you quickly identify any GI complaint.

Create Effective Mnemonics

If you have photographic memory, skip this section. For the rest of us mere mortals, below outlines the organizing principles of what constitutes a Gunner mnemonic.

Mnemonics are important when
1. You have to learn a lot of material.
2. You want to teach something to your colleagues during morning rounds. Attendings and residents are always impressed when they can learn something from a medical student.
3. You want to remember something 15 years from now when you are working the 30th hour of a busy call day. Organizing principles (OP) for mnemonics are as follows:
1. Use the spelling of a name to your benefit (**Spell**) Example:

    a. "8urk14tt's" lymphoma (Burkitt's lymphoma), lep"thin" (leptin), "supraoptiuretic" nuclei (supraoptic nuclei that produce antidiuretic hormone)

    b. Tenofovir is the only NRTI nucleoTide

    c. We"C"ener's granulomatosis (GPA) for C-ANCA and Cyclophosphamide tx

2. Create an acronym that contains distinguishing syllables or letters of names (**Distinguish**)
   Example:

   a. Chronic Alcoholics Steal PhenPhen and Nevar Rifuse Grisee Carbs (<u>Chronic alcohol</u> abuse + <u>St. John</u>'s wort + <u>phen</u>ytoin + <u>pheno</u>barb + <u>nevar</u>ipine + <u>rif</u>ampin + <u>grise</u>ofulvin + <u>carb</u>amazepine)
      - Reinforce mnemonic by spelling name of item-to-be-memorized accordingly
         - For example, "Refus"ampin, "Never"apine, "Greasy"ofulvin, "Carb"amazepine, etc.
      - This ties mnemonic OP 1 with mnemonic OP 2

3. Drawings help (**Draw**)
   Example: Trisomy 13 looks like polydactyly + cleft lip when the number 13 is rotated 90 degrees clockwise (the horizontal 1 is the extra digit, and the cleft of the horizontal 3 is the cleft lip)

4. Counting the letters of a word (**Count**)
   Example: Patau syndrome = 13 letters = Trisomy 13

5. Arrange acronym in alphabetical order (**Arrange**)
   Example: ABCDEF for diphtheria (ADP ribosylation, beta prophage, C Diphtheria, elongation factor 2)
   Examples of instructors who practice this concept well are Dr. John Barone of Kaplan and Dr. Husain Sattar of Pathoma.
   On the flip side, here are examples of poor mnemonics (although you may remember them now given how they were highlighted in this text)

   a. Blind as a bat, mad as a hatter, red as a beet, hot as Hades, dry as a bone, the bowel and bladder lose their tone, and the heart runs alone = poor mnemonic for anticholinergic syndrome
      - This mnemonic forces you to memorize extra and extraneous things (like bat, beet, hare, and desert) which have nothing to do with anticholinergic syndrome.

   b. WWHHHHIMP (withdrawal + Wernicke + hypertensive crisis + hypoxia + hypoglycemia + hypoperfusion + intracranial bleed + meningitis/encephalopathy + poisoning) = poor mnemonic for causes of delirium
      - Wait how many H's does this mnemonic have again?

MNEMONIC

Trisomy 13 mnemonic

A good rule of thumb: if you can still remember a mnemonic under a high-pressure situation (attending pimps you) or after a 7-day period, then you have a winner.

Ultimately, the best mnemonics are the ones you invent and apply repeatedly. So use these mnemonic principles to give yourself a solid head start.

Devise a Study Schedule and Stick to It

The third most important piece of advice for the shelf is to create a study schedule at the beginning of the rotation and follow it. Rotations such as Family Medicine can be draining. Oftentimes you may find yourself coming home after a long clinic day not wanting to study. However, if you are mentally committed to following a schedule, you will find creative ways to get studying done. For example, some students wake up an hour early to read before clinics. Other students fit study material into their white coat and read during downtime. Family Medicine is unique because you likely will not have to take call and have nights and weekends free for study. Try to get a sense from older students how much time you'll have free per week and allocate your time to reading and doing questions accordingly.

Distinguish Rotation-Knowledge From Shelf-Knowledge

Many of the things you learn on your family medicine rotation do not apply to the shelf exam and vice versa. For example, you may be able to impress your Family Medicine attending by committing dosages of asthma medications to memory, but be aware that this will never be a test question on the shelf.

Thus, be able to compartmentalize. Know exactly what is needed for your Family Medicine rotation and what is expected on the shelf to save yourself precious study time. Also, be aware of what patients you are exposed to on your rotation. For instance, if your preceptor only sees geriatric patients in the community, adapt by doing more questions about pediatric patients and skipping over readings about geriatric-related illnesses during study.

IV. Intro to the National Board of Medical Examiners Clinical Science Family Medicine Subject Exam

99 AR

NBME Shelf Exam Website

The Clinical Science Family Medicine NBME Shelf Exam is a unique exam in that it could be 90, 100, or 110 questions long depending on the choice of your clerkship director. The NBME has a "Core 90-item exam" that is all encompassing and reflects the NBME content outline in terms of content distribution. There are two additional 10-question modules, however, that can be added to test "Musculoskeletal/Sports-related injury" and/or "Chronic care." The MSK module focuses on the "diagnosis and management of common musculoskeletal problems) and can bump the MSK content distribution from 5%–10% to 15%–20%. Similarly, the Chronic Care module will have questions that "emphasize continuity of care" of chronic illnesses that may afflict patients across the age continuum (childhood, adolescence, adulthood, and geriatric).

If the Family Medicine shelf is required, make sure to clarify with your clerkship director which modules, if any, will be added to the 90-item core exam. If the MSK module is added, spend more time perusing Chapter 14 of this book. If the Chronic care module is added, focus more on diseases that last across multiple age groups, such as asthma or inflammatory bowel disorder.

Unlike step 1, shelf exam questions focus almost exclusively on disease processes rather than normal processes. However, be familiar with normal aging and development of the child.

According to the NBME, the exams are curved to a mean of 70 with a standard deviation of 8. The curve does not take into account timing of rotation. For instance, students who take the exam during their first block will be held to the same statistical standard as students who take the exam during their fourth clerkship block. However, the NBME does release "quarterly norm information" to medical schools in order to make clerkship directors aware of the relationship between exam score and rotation timing. Importantly, as of now, shelf exam scores are sent to the school directly; students cannot request their shelf exam score independent of their school.

Although different Family Medicine clerkships have different standards for determining grades, in general, each program has its own internally generated shelf exam cutoff score one needs to achieve in order to be eligible for the highest clerkship grade (e.g., Honors). If this is the case, confirm the cutoff score with your clerkship director so that you have a reasonable performance goal to shoot for.

Students are expected to master content organized into these following categories:

System

General Principles, Including Normal Age-Related Findings and Care of the Well Patient	5%–10%
Immune System	1%–5%
Blood and Lymphoreticular System	1%–5%
Behavioral Health	5%–10%
Nervous System and Special Senses	1%–5%
Skin and Subcutaneous Tissue	3%–7%
Musculoskeletal System (% increases with the addition of the Musculoskeletal module)	5%–10%
Cardiovascular System	5%–10%
Respiratory System	5%–10%
Gastrointestinal System	5%–10%
Renal and Urinary System	1%–5%
Pregnancy, Childbirth, and the Puerperium	1%–5%
Female Reproductive System and Breast	1%–5%
Male Reproductive System	1%–5%
Endocrine System	5%–10%
Multisystem Processes and Disorders	1%–5%
Biostatistics, Epidemiology/Population Health, and Interpretation of the Medical Lit.	1%–5%
Social Sciences	5%–10%
Communication and interpersonal skills	
Medical ethics and jurisprudence	
Systems-based practice and patient safety	

Currently, the NBME Clinical Famiiy Medicine Content Outline breaks down question types into three categories

Family Medicine Outline

- Health Maintenance, Prevention, and Surveillance (20%–25%)
- Diagnosis: Including Foundational Science Concepts (40%–50%)
- Pharmacotherapy, Intervention, and Management (25%–30%)

However, devising a study plan from these three categories can be confusing. "Foundational Science Concepts," for instance, is vague and difficult to prepare for. Instead, many students prefer to study according to Physician Tasks provided in older content outlines. Since every subject exam question asks about one of four things – 1) protocol for promoting health maintenance (Prophylaxis [PPx]), 2) the mechanism of disease (MoD), 3) steps to establishing a diagnosis (Dx), and 4) steps of disease management (Tx/Mgmt) – we recommend studying according to Physician Tasks from the 2016 Content Outline.

Physician Tasks (from 2016 Content Outline)

Promoting health and health maintenance	15%–20%
Understanding mechanisms of disease	5%–10%
Establishing a diagnosis	30%–35%
Applying principles of management	25%–30%

In addition, the NBME breaks down questions by Site of Care,

- Ambulatory (60%–65%)
- Emergency Department (25%–30%)
- Inpatient (5%–15%)

And by Patient Age:

- Birth to 17 (10%–15%)
- 18 to 65 (55%–65%)
- 66 and older (20%–25%)
- Our recommendation is to not worry about site of care or age; instead, focus on studying content related to Physician Tasks

Lastly, the distribution of questions according to age groups is as follows:

Distribution Across Age Groups

Birth to 17	15%–20%
18 to 65	55%–65%
66 and older	15%–20%

Gunner Goggles Family Medicine presents material to reflect how the NBME structures its shelf exams. Each chapter that follows falls into the main testable categories of General Principles (Chapter 2) or Organ Systems (Chapter 3–15). Each disease is presented in a "PPx, MoD, Dx and Tx/Mgmt" format, which represents the four physician tasks the NBME can test you on. Since establishing a diagnosis is weighted especially heavily (30%–35%), the "Buzz words" category shows readers how to quickly identify the disease process from just a few key words. The "Clinical Presentation" section serves to more thoroughly describe the disease. However, it is important to note that Buzz Words are sufficient in correctly identifying the corresponding disease on the shelf. The detail provided in the Clinical Presentation section is only meant to augment your understanding, particularly if it is your first pass and you are unfamiliar with the material. However, by the end of studying, the focus should primarily be on Buzz Words.

Finally, here are four things to keep in mind when studying for the Family Medicine shelf:

1. Review the health maintenance guidelines as put out by the American Academy of Family Physicians (AAFP).
2. If pressed for time, practice identifying disease processes only through "Buzz words." For instance, a young adult patient who presents with polyuria, polydipsia, and polyphagia most likely has diabetes.
3. In addition, "Promoting Health and Maintenance" is going to be up to 20 questions so make sure you know your screening guidelines well (e.g., the PPx for each disease presented).
4. Make sure to begin doing questions early (e.g., 10 questions a day starting from day 1). Ideally you should make a second pass of the most high-yield questions before test day.
5. For each question, write a one-line take home point in an Excel spreadsheet. This makes for quick and easy review in the days leading up to the exam.

If any questions arise while studying, use the *Gunner Goggles* app to access the AR features embedded on each page.

Good luck and happy hunting.

—The Gunner Goggles Team

General Principles

Leo Wang, Hao-Hua Wu, and
Katherine Margo

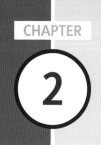

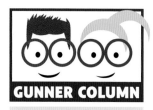

GUNNER COLUMN

Introduction

This chapter is meant to introduce some basic concepts in family medicine that will carry over into many other rotations. It is not meant to be exhaustive, but meant to highlight key points on the family medicine shelf that will be (1) tested and (2) relevant to future shelf exams and (3) relevant to your rotation and practice. We want to emphasize once again that we have distilled this list of general principles from a much longer list that family physicians have to know and thus this chapter will not substitute for your actual rotation experience.

This chapter covers screening and preventative measurements, how to read EKGs, epidemiology, medical ethics, and vitamin deficiencies. Focus particularly on the screening and preventative measurements section and make sure you get a good overview of clinical epidemiology.

Screening, Counseling, Prevention, and Wellness Exams

The following list of topics is high yield and will come up both on the family medicine shelf and as you see patients in real life. These topics are not necessarily diseases and thus are not presented in the traditional Prophylactic (PPx), Mechanism of Disease (MoD), Diagnostic Steps (Dx), and Treatment/Management (Tx/Mgmt) fashion. For more in-depth explorations of the individual diseases, you should refer to specific chapters within the book. These diseases are meant to be an overview of the screening, counseling, and prevention measurements that will come up during a wellness exam for individuals of all ages and genders. Be sure to remember the characteristics of an ideal screening test: one that has a positive result if the patient has the disease and a negative result if the patient does not have the disease. Screening tests are thus a balance between sensitivity and specificity.

Breast Cancer

You should be prepared to counsel your patients on the risk factors for breast cancer and understand the utility of the breast exam. Your family medicine shelf will test your ability to convey these risk factors and the utility of the breast exam to your patients.

- Risk factors:
  - First-degree relative with breast cancer
  - Early menarche or late menopause → increased estrogen exposure
    - Late menarche or early menopause → decreased risk
  - BRCA1/2
  - Age
  - Gender (F>>M)
  - Hormone/radiation therapy
  - Obesity
  - Diethylsilbestrol
  - Late age pregnancies
    - Early pregnancies → decreased risk
  - Breast exam
    - US Preventive Services Task Force (USPTSF) does NOT recommend self breast exams
    - American Cancer Society (ACS) recommends CLINICAL BREAST EXAM every 3 years from age 20 to 39 and every year after age 40
    - USPSTF recommends biennial mammograms after the age of 50

Cervical Cancer

Be prepared to counsel your patients on the risk factors for cervical cancer and the human papillomavirus (HPV) vaccine.

- Risk factors:
  - Early intercourse
  - Increased sexual partners
  - DES exposure
  - Cigarettes
  - Immunosuppression (since caused by HPV?)
- HPV vaccine:
  - Gardasil: HPV 6,11,16, 18 for females age 9–26
  - Cervarix: HPV 16, 18, 31, 45 for males and females aged 10–25
  - All girls and boys aged 11–18 should be vaccinated
  - All vaccines are a series of two or three shots

Menopause

Patients will ask about the definition of menopause, which is defined as the period when ovulation stops because of complete oocyte depletion. The **average** age of menopause is 52, although women aged 40–60 can go through

QUICK TIPS
USPSTF and ACS have different recommendations for breast cancer screening. The USPSTF guidelines are more conservative and likely to decrease the number of false positive results.

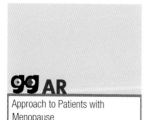

AR

Approach to Patients with
Menopause

it. Menopause is defined as the absence of periods for 12 months and can occur earlier in smokers. The following are symptoms: vaginal dryness, hot flashes, night sweats, sleep disturbances, thinning hair, weight gain, mood changes. Be prepared to explain the symptoms, cause, and also counsel your patient on management. Good practice includes encouraging a healthy lifestyle, smoking cessation and the consideration of hormone therapy in the early 50s.

Perimenopause

Occurs 2–8 years before menopause and the hallmark feature is menstrual irregularity. Other symptoms include hot flashes, vaginal dryness, changes in libido, mood swings. Symptoms of concern include periods being close together, heavy bleeding, spotting, or periods longer than a week. This should raise your suspicion for other pathologies.

Osteoporosis

Osteoporosis is a concern for all women especially after menopause. Be able to counsel your patients on the risk factors. Be able to counsel your patients on regular exercise especially WEIGHT-BEARING, adequate nutrition, and smoking/alcohol cessation. Pharmacologic treatment includes raloxifene or bisphosphonates. The FRAX score can be used to classify osteoporotic patients.

- Risk factors:
  - Low estrogen (late menarche, early menopause)
  - Inadequate physical activity
  - Body mass index (BMI)
  - Inadequate calcium
  - Family history
  - Cigarettes
  - Dementia
  - History of fractures
- DEXA screening:
  - BMI > 30
    - High estrogen level, protective against menopausal symptoms and osteoporosis
  - USPSTF: evidence is insufficient for or against screening in postmenopausal women younger than 60
  - USPSTF recommends screening DEXA in all women over 65, and all women 60–64 with increased fracture risk

FOR THE WARDS

Low estrogen → osteoporosis but prevents against breast cancer. High estrogen → breast cancer but prevents against osteoporosis. It's a catch-22!

Obesity

Obesity is an epidemic in the United States. Recognize the complications of obesity, how to use the BMI, and how to counsel patients to lose weight and encourage a healthier lifestyle.

- Complications of obesity:
  - Insulin resistance, elevated cholesterol, triglycerides
  - Type 2 diabetes mellitus (DM), hypertension (HTN), CHD, stroke, peripheral vascular disease, polycystic ovary syndrome (PCOS)
  - Congestive heart failure (CHF), AFib, Gout, OA, chronic back pain, deep vein thrombosis (DVTs), gallstones, gastroesophageal reflux disease (GERD)
  - Obesity in women → irregular menses, anovulation, infertility
  - BMI > 40 increases risk of cancer
- Obesity diagnosis from BMI:
  - BMI calculation:
    - weight (in kilograms)/height (in meters) squared
    - weight (in pounds)/height (in inches) squared × 703 height (in inches) squared
      - BMI: 26–30 is overweight, >30 is obese, <18.5 is underweight
      - Obesity: more than 30–35 is class I, 35–40 is class II, more than 40 is class III or morbid obesity
- Management:
  - 3500 calorie deficit → 1 pound of weight loss
  - Aim to lose half a pound to a pound a week
  - Focus on diet and exercise
    - 30 minutes a day of moderate exercise most days OR 20 minutes if vigorous exercise 3 days a week
      - Moderate: 50%–70% of MAX HR (220-age)
      - Always ask about lifestyle and interests, get patient motivation, incorporate physical activity into things they already do
  - Consider pharmacologic intervention for patients BMI >30:
    - Orlistat
    - Phentermine/Topamax
    - Bariatric surgery

99 AR

AAFP Medical Management of Obesity

Immunizations

Know the current recommendations about TdaP, HPV, pneumonia, and flu shots for adults, as well as recommendations for adolescents and college students. Immunization schedules are recommended by the CDC. See http://www.cdc.gov/vaccines/schedules/hcp/index.html for the schedules (Figs. 2.1 and 2.2).

These recommendations must be read with the footnotes that follow. For those who fall behind or start late, provide catch-up vaccination at the earliest opportunity as indicated by the green bars in Figure 1. To determine minimum intervals between doses, see the catch-up schedule (Figure 2). School entry and adolescent vaccine age groups are shaded.

Vaccine	Birth	1 mo	2 mos	4 mos	6 mos	9 mos	12 mos	15 mos	18 mos	19–23 mos	2–3 yrs	4–6 yrs	7–10 yrs	11–12 yrs	13–15 yrs	16–18 yrs
Hepatitis B[1] (HepB)	1st dose	←2nd dose→			←——————— 3rd dose ———————→											
Rotavirus[2] (RV) RV1 (2-dose series); RV5 (3-dose series)			1st dose	2nd dose	See footnote 2											
Diphtheria, tetanus, & acellular pertussis[3] (DTaP: <7 yrs)			1st dose	2nd dose	3rd dose		←———— 4th dose ————→					5th dose				
Haemophilus influenzae type b[4] (Hib)			1st dose	2nd dose	See footnote 4		3rd or 4th dose, See footnote 4									
Pneumococcal conjugate[5] (PCV13)			1st dose	2nd dose	3rd dose		←—— 4th dose ——→									
Inactivated poliovirus[6] (IPV: <18 yrs)			1st dose	2nd dose	←——————— 3rd dose ———————→							4th dose				
Influenza[7] (IIV; LAIV)						Annual vaccination (IIV only) 1 or 2 doses					Annual vaccination (LAIV or IIV) 1 or 2 doses		Annual vaccination (LAIV or IIV) 1 dose only			
Measles, mumps, rubella[8] (MMR)							←———— 1st dose ————→					2nd dose				
Varicella[9] (VAR)							←———— 1st dose ————→					2nd dose				
Hepatitis A[10] (HepA)							←——— 2-dose series, See footnote 10 ———→									
Meningococcal[11] (Hib-MenCY ≥ 6 weeks; MenACWY-D ≥9 mos; MenACWY-CRM ≥ 2 mos)							See footnote 11							1st dose		Booster
Tetanus, diphtheria, & acellular pertussis[12] (Tdap: ≥7yrs)														(Tdap)		
Human papillomavirus[13] (2vHPV: females only; 4vHPV, 9vHPV: males and females)														(3-dose series)		
Meningococcal B[11]														See footnote 11		
Pneumococcal polysaccharide[5] (PPSV23)													See footnote 5			

Legend:
- Range of recommended ages for all children
- Range of recommended ages for catch-up immunization
- Range of recommended ages for certain high-risk groups
- Range of recommended ages for non-high-risk groups that may receive vaccine, subject to individual clinical decision making
- No recommendation

FIG. 2.1 Recommended immunization schedule for persons aged 0–18 years–United States, 2016. (FOR THOSE WHO FALL BEHIND OR START LATE, SEE THE CATCH-UP SCHEDULE [see Fig. 2.2]).

VACCINE ▼ AGE GROUP ▶	19-21 years	22-26 years	27-49 years	50-59 years	60-64 years	≥65 years
Influenza[*,2]	1 dose annually					
Tetanus, diphtheria, pertussis (Td/Tdap)[*,3]	Substitute Tdap for Td once, then Td booster every 10 yrs					
Varicella[*,4]	2 doses					
Human papillomavirus (HPV) Female[*,5]	3 doses					
Human papillomavirus (HPV) male[*,5]	3 doses					
Zoster[6]					1 dose	
Measles, mumps, rubella (MMR)[*,7]	1 or 2 doses depending on indication					
Pneumococcal 13-valent conjugate (PCV13)[*,8]						1 dose
Pneumococcal 23-valent polysaccharide (PPSV23)[8]	1 or 2 doses depending on indication					1 dose
Hepatitis A[*,9]	2 or 3 doses depending on vaccine					
Hepatitis B[*,10]	3 doses					
Meningococcal 4-valent conjugate (MenACWY) or polysaccharide (MPSV4)[*,11]	1 or more doses depending on indication					
Meningococcal B (MenB)[11]	2 or 3 doses depending on vaccine					
Haemophilus influenzae type b (Hib)[*,12]	1 or 3 doses depending on indication					

*Covered by the vaccine injury compensation program

Recommended for all persons who meet the age requirement, lack documentation of vaccination, or lack evidence of past infection; zoster vaccine is recommended regardless of past episode of zoster

Recommended for persons with a risk factor (medical, occupational, lifestyle, or other indication)

No recommendation

Report all clinically significant postvaccination reactions to the vaccine adverse event reporting system (VAERS). Reporting forms and instructions on filing a VAERS report are available at www.vaers.hhs.gov or by telephone, 800-822-7967.

Information on how to file a vaccine injury compensation program claim is available at www.hrsa.gov/vaccinecompensation or by telephone, 800-338-2382. To file a claim for vaccine injury, contact the U.S. court of Federal Claims, 717 Madison place, N.W., Washington, D.C. 20005; telephone, 202-357-6400.

Additional information about the vaccines in schedule, extent of available data, and contraindications for vaccination is also available at www.cdc.gov/vaccines or from the CDC-INFO contact center at 800-CDC-INFO (800-232-4636) in english and spanish, 8:00 a.m. - 8:00 p.m. Eastern Time, Monday - Friday, excluding holidays.

Use of trade names and commercial sources is for identification only and does not imply endorsement by the U.S. department of health and human services.

The recommendations in this schedule were approved by the centers for disease control and prevention's (CDC) advisory committee on immunization practices (ACIP), the american academy of family physicians (AAFP), the america college of physicians (ACP), the american college of obstetricians and gynecologists (ACOG) and the american college of nurse-midwives (ACNM).

FIG. 2.2 Recommended immunization schedule for adults aged 19 years or older, by vaccine and age group.[1]

Cardiovascular Disease

Screening for cardiovascular disease is covered in Chapter 7. Cardiovascular disease is the leading cause of mortality in the United States. Make no mistake that this is an incredibly important section on the family medicine shelf. Make sure patients know the risk factors:

- Sedentary
- Tobacco
- Alcohol
- Stress
- Diet
- Obesity
- Old age
- Male gender
- Family history

Smoking

Smoking is a major problem with many complications. Be sure you can counsel your patients on the complications in addition to smoking cessation.

- Smoking complications:
  - Lung cancer and others (bladder)
  - CHD
  - COPD
  - GERD
  - Gingivitis
  - Damages babies

Tobacco addiction is characterized by **3 Cs: Compulsion, lack of Control, and Continued use** despite adverse circumstance. In counseling patients on tobacco cessation, recognize the phases of behavior change: pre-contemplative, contemplative, active, relapse.

- Management of Smoking Cessation—5 As:
  - Ask or address behavior
  - Assess interest
  - Advice on methods
  - Assist with motivation
  - Arrange for follow-up

Oral medications can be effective (1.5–3 times placebo in a year)

- Most smokers quit many times before actual success
  - Quit rates: 2%–3% per year
- Groups improve quit rates
- One-on-one counseling enhances quitting success but only when **combined with medication**

When patient is ready to quit smoking:

1. Set a date

2. Go to 1-800-QUITNOW or Smokefree.gov
3. Instruct patient to take bupropion or varenicline 1 week before quitting
   - One pill per day for first 3 days, then one pill twice per day for next 4 days. Then quit smoking, and keep taking one pill twice a day.
   - May add nicotine gum for bad cravings if needed
   - Stop after 2 months.

The USPSTF recommends annual screening for lung cancer with low-dose computed tomography (CT) in those aged 55–80 with a 30-pack per year history and either currently smoke or quit within 15 years, although this is somewhat controversial.

Alcohol

Many of your patients will consume alcohol. Use the CAGE questionnaire to assess their dependency.
- CAGE:
  - Cut down?
  - Annoyed?
  - Guilty?
  - Eye opener?
  - If any of these are yes, further questions are necessary

Nutritional Counseling

- Brief history for diet should include:
  - number of meals and snacks in a 24-hour period
  - dining-out habits
  - frequency of fruits, vegetables, meats, poultry, fish, dairy products and desserts consumed
- For complete dietary history:
  - 24-hour dietary recall on each meal
  - **WAVE:** pocket card designed to encourage dialogue about the patient's:
    - Weight
    - Activity
    - Variety
    - Excess
  - Food frequency questionnaire: covers food intake over period of a month; used in combination with 24-hour recall, it is the quickest way to determine nutritional deficiencies and excesses.
  - Dietary intake records (food diaries): ask patient to bring in complete record of everything over 3–4 day period.

Prostate Cancer

- USPSTF recommends against PSA screening.
- ACS and AUA recommend testing to men at age 50, but physician should first discuss risks and harms.
- Benefits:
  - Psychological reassurance with negative screen or of detecting cancer at a treatable stage
- Potential harms:
  - Pain and discomfort with prostate biopsy
  - Psychological effects of false-positives
  - Complications from treatment of cancer that may not have caused symptoms

Colon Cancer

- Methods:
  - Direct visualization with colonoscopy every 10 years from 50 to 75 years old; 76–85 years old on a case-by-case basis
  - Fecal Immunochemical Test (FIT), guaiac fecal occult blood test (gFOBT) or FIT-DNA every year as stool-based tests
  - Flexible sigmoidoscopy every 10 years with FIT every year (visualization and stool-based combination)
  - Insufficient evidence about CT colonography

99 AR

Life years gained per 1000 individuals screened

Exercise Prescription

The key is to give specific recommendations.
- Type of activity
  - Patient preference; swimming or water jogging is better for those with arthritis
- Precautions: orthopedic consult if needed?
- Specific workloads?
- Duration and frequency
  - For fitness, 30 minutes three times a week—current recommendation is 150 minutes/week
  - Weight loss, 20–30 minutes a day
- Intensity
  - Target heart rate (THR) 220 − age × 0.7–0.8
  - THR is related to rate of perceived exertion (RPE); should be about a 12–24/20 on the **Borg scale**

Well Child Exam

A good well-child exam should include a history and physical.
- History
- PE

- Height, weight, BMI, blood pressure (BP)—make sure to check against age related parameters
- Ophthalmic exam
  - Pupillary light reflex, test for strabismus
  - Vision
- Mouth
  - Dental caries, gingival inflammation
- Neurologic
  - Fine/gross motor skill exam
  - Language, speech, clarity, thought content
  - Hearing
- There are **no contraindications** to immunization on the family medicine shelf unless there is a blatant, life-threatening allergy.

Biostatics and Epidemiology for the Family Medicine Shelf

The family medicine shelf will test your biostatistics capacity. This is the same material that you learned for step 1. If you remember your stats from step 1 (e.g., sensitivity, specificity, NPV, PPV, OR, RR, ARR, type 1 and 2 error, null hypothesis), feel free to skip this section. Otherwise spend no more than 30 minutes reviewing the material below (Tables 2.1 and 2.2).

Finally, understand the basics behind statistical testing. Anytime you run a statistical test, you are determining if there is or is not a relationship between two variables. For example, is there a relationship between smoking and lung cancer? Yes. Is there a relationship between a positive pregnancy test and lung cancer? No. Is there a relationship between a positive pregnancy test and pregnancy? Yes. Do men weigh more than women? Yes. Statistical testing is the way we are able to say yes, no, yes and yes to the previous questions with some amount of certainty, although any real statistician will tell you that you cannot say anything with absolute certainty in statistics.

Your null hypothesis is a statement you make where you assume no relationship between two variables you are testing. For example, your null hypothesis could be that smoking does not cause lung cancer, or that sex does not influence weight. You then run some kind of statistical test that will assess that relationship. You will only need to know two for the family medicine shelf.

1. T-test tests whether two variables are from the same group or from different groups. Imagine that the average weight of men is 150 and average weight of

TABLE 2.1 Diagnostic Tests

		DISEASE	
		+	−
Test	+	TP (patients with disease, test positive)	FP (patients without disease, test positive)	PPV = TP/(TP+FP)
	−	FN (patients with disease, test negative)	TN (patients without disease, test negative)	NPV = TN/(TN+FN)
	−	Sensitivity = TP/(TP+FN)	Specificity = TN/(TN+FP)	−

Sensitivity—how many people who have the disease will test positive?
= true positives/(total who test positive for disease)
– Total who test positive for disease = false positive (people who don't have disease but actually test positive falsely) and true positive (people who have disease and test positive)
= true positives/(false positives + true positives)
Specificity—how many people who don't have the disease will test negative?
= true negatives/(total who test negative for disease)
– People who test negative for disease = false negative (people who actually have the disease and test falsely negative) and true negative (people who don't have the disease and test negative)
= true negatives/(false negatives + true negatives)
Positive predictive value—how many people who test positive actually have the disease?
= true positives/(total people who have the disease)
– Total people who have the disease = true positives (have disease, test positive) and false negatives (have disease, test falsely negative)
= true positives/(true positive + false negative)
Negative predictive value—how many people who test negative actually don't have the disease?
= true negatives/(total people who don't have the disease)
– Total people who don't have disease = true negatives (don't have disease, test negative) and false positives (don't have disease, test falsely positive)
= true negatives/(true negatives + false positives)
FN, False negative; *FP*, false positive; *NPV*, negative predictive value; *PPV*, positive predictive value; *TN*, test negative; *TP*, test negative.

women is 100. Your t-test here would find these two averages come from different groups; another way of rephrasing this is that your sex influences your weight and the two variables are related. Here, you would reject the null hypothesis if and only if $P < .05$. We discuss this later.

2. An ANOVA tests whether several variables are from the same group or from different groups. Imagine that the average blood pressure of construction workers is 140, doctors is 120, nurses is 130, lawyers is 110, and that astronauts is 210 (this is absolutely not true, by the way). Your ANOVA would find that astronauts have a much higher blood pressure than the other groups. Another way of saying this would be that your occupation influences your blood pressure. Here, you would again reject the null hypothesis under specific conditions (Bonferroni correction) that are not relevant to the family medicine shelf.

TABLE 2.2 Risk Factor Versus Disease

		DISEASE	
		+	−
Risk factor	+	A	B
OR	−	C	D
Intervention			

This is the only thing used in case control studies:
Odds Ratio (OR): Only used in case control studies, odds of being exposed to risk factor in patients with disease divided by odds of being exposed to risk factor in patients without disease

$$OR = (a/c)/(b/d)$$

Everything else is used in cohort studies:
Relative Risk (RR): Only used in cohort studies, risk of getting disease in patients with risk factor divided by risk of getting disease in patients without risk factor

$$RR = [a/(a+b)]/[c/(c+d)]; \text{ relative risk reduction} = 1 - RR$$

Attributable Risk (AR, risk gain): Only used in cohort studies looking at a negative exposure (i.e., smoking for lung cancer), risk of getting disease in patients with risk factor minus risk of getting disease in patients without risk factor

$$AR = a/(a+b) - c/(c+d); \text{ number needed to harm} = 1/AR$$

Absolute Risk Reduction (ARR, risk loss): Only used in cohort studies looking at a positive exposure or preventative measure (i.e., exercise for MI), risk of getting disease in patients without preventative measure − risk of getting disease in patients with preventative measure

$$ARR = c/(c+d) - a/(a+b); \text{ number needed to treat} = 1/ARR$$

Every statistical test requires you to pick an alpha threshold that you are comfortable with. Most people pick 0.05, or 5%. Alpha is your chance of making a type I error, (stating there is a difference when one does not really exist, or erroneously ejecting the null)—put simply, it's your odds of finding a relationship and not being wrong about it, or your odds of getting a false positive result. The p-value your statistical test gives you is the odds of a type I error. The lower the better, and the more likely it is you can actually reject your null hypothesis without committing a type I error. For example, if I were to receive a p-value of 0.01 from a statistical test between the weights of men and women, I would conclude there is only a 1% chance that we committed a type I error if I reject the mean. That means if we run this test 99 times, we would get the same result 99 times and only 1 of those times would we actually have incorrectly rejected the null. Put simply, it means that we have a 99% chance of finding this same relationship (sex influences weight) if we did the test again. Conversely, if we got a p value of 0.5 or 50%, this means that there is a 50% chance that if we did this test again that we would get a different

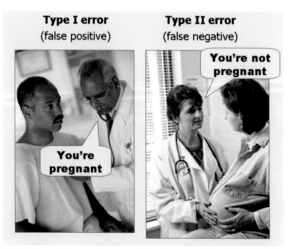

FIG. 2.3 Remember, we're more willing to accept type II errors than type I errors from statistical testing, but we really shouldn't be making either!

relationship—thus, half the time sex influences weight, the other half of the time it doesn't. We wouldn't be able to conclude that sex influences weight here!

The other concept that relates closely to alpha is beta. Beta is the opposite of the alpha, and is the likelihood of accepting the null when there is a real relationship. This is a type II error: the odds of you actually concluding that positive pregnancy tests have no relationship with pregnancy, when in reality there is an obvious relationship. While alpha is set at very low thresholds like 0.05, beta is usually set around 0.2. This means that we are okay with as high of a 20% chance of making a type II error, whereas we set alpha at much lower. Why? It's because false negatives are bad, but false positives are even worse. We want to be able to trust the results of a positive statistical test more than we want to be able to trust the results of a negative one; if our positive tests were getting a bunch of false positive measurements, they'd be meaningless. Remember beta is influenced by three things: sample size, effect size, and precision of measurement. Increasing all of the aforementioned will decrease beta, and decrease odds of a type II error (Fig. 2.3).

Medical Ethics for the Family Medicine Shelf

Patient characteristics associated with adherence can appear on any shelf exam and family medicine is fair game. Learn what to do and not to do in the following ethical scenarios. These concepts test your mastery of building the patient-doctor relationship, the strength of which is most closely related to patient adherence. In general, think how your doctoring or doctor-patient preceptor/mentor would respond and answer accordingly. The safest answer is usually correct. When in doubt, prioritize the patient's autonomy and comfort first and foremost.

1. Patient with suicidal ideation
   Action: Assess threat (e.g., detailed plan vs. passing thought); if threat is serious (e.g., detailed plan, consistent suicidal ideation), make sure patient is admitted to hospital voluntarily or involuntarily. Patients may be held involuntarily if threat to self or others.
   Avoid: Assuming threat is not serious, question stem may contain fillers to obfuscate severity of SI admission.

2. Patient nonadherent to treatment or test
   Action: Ask why patient is nonadherent and be respectful.
   Avoid: Referring patient to another physician.

3. Patient nonadherent to total lifestyle change, behavior
   Action: Ask about patient's willingness to change behavior. If patient is not willing, then provider cannot move on to next step why and issue needs to be addressed.
   Avoid: Forcing patient to change if not willing to or scaring patient.

4. Patient who is seductive
   Action: Set limits, define tolerable behavior, see patient with chaperone.
   Avoid: Refusing to care for patient, asking open-ended questions, referring patient to another physician, entering into relationship with patient (never the right answer).

5. Patient who is angry
   Action: NURSE: Name the emotion (e.g., "You appear angry."). Understand why and thank patient for sharing. Recognize what patient is doing right. Show support for the patient. Explore emotion.
   Avoid: Taking patient's anger personally.

6. Patient who is sad and tearful
   Action: NURSE: Name the emotion (e.g., "You appear angry."). Understand why and thank patient for sharing. Recognize what patient is doing right. Show support for the patient. Explore emotion.

Avoid: Using patronizing statements such as "do not worry," rushing patient, and stating "I understand." instead, further explore emotion to better understand where patient is coming from.

7. Patient who complains about another doctor

Action: Recommend patient speak to other doctor directly.

Avoid: Saying anything to disparage the other doctor, intervening with care unless emergent need.

8. Patient who complains about you or your staff

Action: Verify complaint, speak to staff member who was named in complaint.

Avoid: Blaming patient, being defensive.

9. Patient who you need to break bad news to

Action: SPIKES: Set-up patient encounter by making sure patient is sitting in a chair with social support nearby. Ask about patient perception of what is going on. Ask patient for an invitation or permission to share the bad news. Explain your own knowledge of the bad news; make sure to preface by statements that convey the gravity of the situation (e.g., "I'm worried" or "I have bad news"). Manage patient's emotion after bad news is shared. Summarize situation and suggest concrete next steps.

Avoid: Sharing bad news when patient is in a vulnerable position (e.g., standing up while on the phone), breaking bad news without warning.

10. Patient being evaluated for decision-making capacity

Action: Determine if patient meets criteria for being a legally competent decision-maker, including (1) patients ≥18 or legally emancipated through marriage, military or financial independence; (2) patient makes and communicates a choice; (3) patient knows and understands benefit and risks; (4) patient decision stable over time; (5) decision congruent to patient value system; (6) decision not a result of mood disorder, hallucinations, or delusions. Patients with adequate decision-making capacity can refuse labs, imaging (e.g., CT scans), and treatment.

Avoid: Assuming patient lacks decision-making capacity if <18 (remember marriage, military and financial independence from parents).

11. Patient who is a Jehovah's witness and needs blood transfusion

Action: Determine if patient meets criteria for not needing informed consent (e.g., legally incompetent, implied consent in emergency with no ability for communication, patient waived right to informed consent).

Avoid: Giving blood if patient does not give consent but not meet one of the exceptions.

12. Patient with meningitis refusing treatment

Action: Determine if patient has right to refuse treatment; in this case, patient does not have a right because doing so would pose a threat to the health and welfare of others.

Avoid: Consulting hospital ethics committee unless there is a dilemma with no clear way to proceed.

13. Pediatric patient with non-emergent, potentially fatal medical condition and parents refuse treatment

Action: Seek a court order mandating treatment.

Avoid: Complying with parents' demand.

Pediatric patient + non-emergent condition + no parental approval → proceed with treatment only after legal approval granted

14. Patient with HIV diagnosis refuses to share with significant other

Action: Assess confidentiality rules; in this case, significant other needs to be legally notified to prevent harm from transmission. Encourage patient to discuss health and medical conditions with loved ones. Share patient results with local health department.

Avoid: Allowing patient to avoid disclosing potentially fatal communicable disease.

QUICK TIPS

Pediatric patient + emergent condition + no parental approval → proceed with treatment anyway

Vitamin Deficiencies

Vitamin deficiencies are frequently tested on the family medicine shelf. Be able to identify vitamin deficiencies based on the buzz words, and recognize the diagnostic steps in differentiating between them. All vitamin deficiencies occur through supplementation of the missing vitamin, so this basic principle is not frequently tested.

Vitamin A (Retinol) Deficiency

Buzz Words: Night blindness + dry skin + alopecia + corneal degeneration → vitamin A deficiency

PPx: Vitamin A supplementation

MoD: Lack of vitamin A, that is needed to bind a protein in retina, can cause inability to see through dim light at night (night-blindness).

- Deficiency occurs rarely in fat malabsorption syndromes that are caused by cystic fibrosis, biliary atresia, and sprue.

Dx:
1. Clinical symptoms
Tx/Mgmt:
1. Vitamin A supplementation

Vitamin B1 (Thiamine) Deficiency

Buzz Words:
- Peripheral neuropathy w/ symmetric impairment of sensory, motor, and reflex functions → distal > proximal limb segments with calf muscle tenderness → dry beriberi
- Confusion, muscular atrophy, "edema," tachycardia, cardiomegaly, CHF with peripheral neuropathy → wet beriberi
- Alcoholic with retrograde and anterograde amnesia and confabulation (altered mental status, opthalmoplegia, ataxia [AOA]) → Wernicke-Korsakoff syndrome

PPx: None; avoid abusing alcohol
MoD: Thiamine deficiency → catabolism of sugars and amino acids in neurons
Dx:
1. History and physical
Tx/Mgmt:
1. IV infusion of vitamin B1 in the acute stage (Wernicke encephalopathy). In the chronic stage (Korsakoff syndrome), only supportive care can be provided

Vitamin B3 (Niacin; Nicotinic Acid) Deficiency

- Also known as pellagra ("rough skin")

Buzz Words: Diarrhea + dementia + dermatitis→ pellagra
PPx: None
MoD: Decreased NAD production (NAD and its phosphorylated NADP form are cofactors required in many body processes); often from deficiency in tryptophan—occurring in people who only consume corn—lacking nicotinic acid and tryptophan that can be converted into nicotinic acid.
  - Primarily causes symptoms of three organs (gastrointestinal [GI], nervous system, and skin)

Dx:
1. clinical syndrome—diarrhea, skin changes and memory problem/inattention/confusion/spasticity
Tx/Mgmt:
1. Nicotinamide (same structure but lower toxicity)

Vitamin B6 (Pyridoxine) Deficiency

Buzz Words:
- Skin rash, atrophic glossitis with ulceration, angular cheilitis, conjunctivitis, intertrigo, and neurologic

symptoms of somnolence, confusion with sideroblastic anemia in patient with tuberculosis taking isoniazid therapy → B6 (pyridoxine) deficiency
- Seizures in infants (pyridoxine-responsive seizure)

PPx: Vitamin supplementation with isoniazid for patients receiving tuberculosis treatment

MoD: Cofactor in reactions of amino acid, glucose, lipid metabolism → neuropathy from impaired sphingosin synthesis

Dx:
1. H&P ([a] seizures in infants
2. neuropathy in adult patients

Tx/Mgmt:
1. Pyridoxine hydrochloride to replace vitamin B6

Vitamin B12 (Cobalamin) Deficiency

- Also known as subacute combined degeneration of the spinal cord that presents with posterior and lateral column signs.

Buzz Words: Bone marrow promegaloblastosis (megaloblastic anemia from inhibition of purine synthesis), GI symptoms, weakness, spasticity, absent reflexes, diminished vibration and position sensation, subacute degeneration of spinal cord, memory loss, depression → B12 deficiency

PPx: B12 supplementation, diet including animal products

MoD: Decreased B12 → Impaired DNA synthesis and regulation, fatty acid and amino acid metabolism

Dx:
1. Labs → vitamin B12 levels with elevated methylmalonic acid levels
2. anti-intrinsic factor antibodies to r/o pernicious anemia

Tx/Mgmt:
1. Vitamin B12 supplementation

Vitamin D Deficiency

Buzz Words: Adult + bone pain + weakness + poor fracture healing + hypocalcemic tetany → vitamin D deficiency in adults = osteomalacia; prolonged vitamin D deficiency can cause myelopathy—weakness in legs

PPx: Consumption of milk and sun exposure

MoD: Decreased vitamin D → decreased intestinal absorption of calcium and phosphate → decreased bone mineralization

Dx:
1. Serum level of 25-hydroxyvitamin D
2. PTH levels to r/o endocrine disorder

QUICK TIPS

B12 vs. folate deficiency: There are no neurologic symptoms in folate deficiency.

QUICK TIPS

Calcitriol = active form of vitamin D

Tx/Mgmt:
1. Vitamin D supplementation

Vitamin E Deficiency

Buzz Words: Hemolytic anemia + muscle weakness + acanthocytosis + spinocerebellar ataxia + loss of vibratory sensation and proprioception → vitamin E deficiency

PPx: None

MoD: Vitamin E protects cellular membranes and is an antioxidant

Dx:
1. H&P—ataxic gait and weakness in legs

Tx/Mgmt:
1. Supplementation with vitamin E

Vitamin C Deficiency

Buzz Words: Weakness, fatigue + curly hair, dry mouth

PPx: Vitamin C in diet from citrus/fruits/vegetables

MoD: Vitamin C or ascorbic acid accelerates many biochemical processes, especially in the synthesis of collagen.

Dx: Physical exam

Tx/Mgmt: Vitamin C supplementation

Vitamin K Deficiency

Buzz Words: Bleeding

Zinc Deficiency

Buzz Words: Hypogonadism + delayed wound healing + developmental problems + unable to taste, unable to smell + hair loss **+ skin rash**

QUICK TIPS

Cystic fibrosis patients = vitamin E deficiency 2/2 pancreatic dysfunction

QUICK TIPS

Remember, vitamin K = F II, VII, IX, X and protein C/S

QUICK TIPS

Zinc is probably the one vitamin you don't want to be missing out on when out on a date.

GUNNER PRACTICE

1. A 56-year-old man comes in to your clinic for an annual wellness exam. He is currently being managed for hypertension but is otherwise in good health. He has a 10-pack per year smoking history from his 20s, and has one alcoholic drink each evening. His BMI is 32. Which of the following is not indicated for this patient?
   A. Counseling about obesity
   B. Lung cancer screening
   C. Fecal occult blood test
   D. CAGE questionnaire
   E. Influenza immunization

2. A 28-year-old woman comes into your office with her mother to get information about weight loss. Her BMI is

40. Her siblings, mother, and father are all overweight. She has no other co-morbid medical conditions. She asks you about the best approach to her weight loss. Which of the following is the most appropriate management in this patient?
A. Phentermine
B. Bariatric surgery
C. Orlistat
D. Exercise prescription and dietary intervention
E. No intervention necessary

ANSWERS: What Would Gunner Jess/Jim Do?

1. WWGJD? A 56-year-old **man** comes in to your clinic for an annual wellness exam. He is currently being managed for **hypertension** but is otherwise in good health. He has a 10-pack per year smoking history from his 20s, and has one alcoholic drink each evening. His BMI is 32. Which of the following is not indicated for this patient?

Answer: B, Lung cancer screening.

Explanation: There are no indications for lung cancer screening at this moment. The USPSTF recommends annual screening for lung cancer with CT in those aged 55–80 with a 30-pack per year history and either currently smoke or quit within 15 years. This man has not smoked for 15 years, and does not need lung cancer screening. His 10-pack per year history also does not meet criteria.

A. Counseling about obesity → Incorrect. All patients with a BMI over 30 should be counseled about obesity. This patient's BMI is 32 and he should be approached about lifestyle habits.

C. Fecal occult blood test → Incorrect. After age 50, all men should receive one of the colorectal cancer screening tests such as fecal occult blood tests annually as a screening measure for colon cancer.

D. CAGE questionnaire → Incorrect. CAGE questionnaire should be used in this patient to assess alcohol dependence.

E. Influenza immunization → Incorrect. All men should receive the influenza vaccination annually.

2. WWGJD? A 28-year-old **woman** comes into your office with her mother to get information about **weight loss.** Her BMI is 40. Her siblings, mother, and father are all overweight. She has no other co-morbid medical conditions. She asks you about the best approach to her weight loss. Which of the following is the most appropriate management in this patient?

Answer: D, Exercise prescription and dietary intervention

Explanation: →exercise and dietary prescription should always be first line in management for obese or overweight patients. A 3-month trial should be used to see if success can be had before medical or surgical intervention is necessary. The key to successful intervention is **specific** recommendations.

A. Phentermine → incorrect. While phentermine can be used as a pharmacologic treatment for obesity, it should never used as a first-line agent.

B. Bariatric surgery → incorrect. Bariatric surgery has great success for weight loss but is a last resort treatment for patients with BMI > 40.

C. Orlistat → incorrect. While orlistat can be used as a pharmacologic treatment for obesity, it should never be used as a first-line agent.

E. No intervention necessary → incorrect. Someone with a BMI as high as 40 is at great risk for cardiovascular disease and cancer. Counseling is absolutely necessary and treatment plans should be prescribed.

Immunologic Disorders

Leo Wang, Hao-Hua Wu, and Katherine Margo

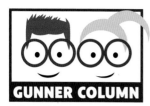

GUNNER COLUMN

Introduction

For the immunologic disorders, know the buzz words for high-yield topics such as hypersensitivity reactions, lupus, and sexually transmitted infections (STIs). In addition, make sure to learn the most commonly tested screening guidelines for STIs, which are included in the prophylactic (PPx) section.

This chapter is divided into (1) immunologically mediated disorders, (2) multisystem infectious disorders, (3) autoimmune disorders, (4) sexually transmitted disorders, and (5) Gunner Practice.

Immunologically Mediated Disorders

Immunologically mediated disorders can be thought of as disease due to an overactive immune response. The actors in the immune system are responding too well to insults. These disorders are high yield for the family medicine subject exams and will appear on other shelfs as well. Hypersensitivity reactions will appear prominently on the Pediatrics shelf and Graft versus host disease will be featured prominently on the Surgery shelf.

TABLE 3.1 Types of Hypersensitivity Reactions: Mechanisms and Examples

Hypersensitivity	Mediated by	Mechanism of Action	Example
Type 1	IgE	Allergen binds and cross links two IgE molecules attached to mast cells	Atopy/ urticaria/ anaphylaxis
Type 2	Antibodies	Antibody attack antigen	ABO incompatibility + Rh hemolytic disease

TABLE 3.1 Types of Hypersensitivity Reactions: Mechanisms and Examples—cont'd

Hypersensitivity	Mediated by	Mechanism of Action	Example
Type 3	Immune complex-mediated	IgG or IgM antibodies form immune complexes → nonspecifically activates inflammatory process	Serum sickness syndrome (antibody-containing-blood mediated) Arthus reaction Serum sickness-like reaction (drug mediated)
Type 4	Cell-mediated (T-cell)	Prior exposure to allergen before developing reaction; reexposure activated cell-mediated response	**Allergic contact dermatitis** from poison ivy, oak, or sumac

Multisystem Infectious Disorders

For bacterial infections, you only need to know buzz words, such as targetoid lesion for Lyme disease. Diagnostic Steps (Dx), Mechanism of Disease (MoD), and Treatment/Management (Tx/Mgmt) are mostly step 1 material. For the shelf exam, it is more likely that you will only have to recognize the disease in the question stem so just look at the buzz words. Rarely will you have to differentiate bacterial versus fungal versus parasitic vs. viral etiology of infection. Instead, it will be obvious from the answer choices that you need to identify a bacterial source of disease, thereby narrowing the differential.

Lyme Disease (*Borrelia burgdorferi*)

Buzz Words: Bilateral Bell's palsy + no other signs of peripheral neuropathy → Lyme disease (be sure to differentiate from Guillain-Barre syndrome, which can present with bilateral Bell's palsy associated with ascending paralysis)
Hiking in tall grass + (late) EKG shows third-degree AV block + joint pain (arthritis) + facial nerve palsy → Lyme disease

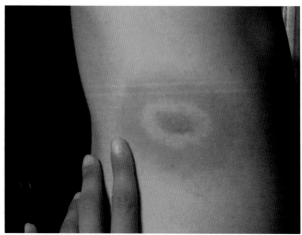

FIG. 3.1 Erythema migrans (characteristic "Bulls-eye" or targetoid lesion). Wikipedia: https://en.wikipedia.org/wiki/Erythema_chronicum_migrans#/media/File:Bullseye_Lyme_Disease_Rash.jpg

Clinical Presentation: This is the most high-yield bacterial infection to know for the shelf because it affects multiple organ systems and can present in a variety of ways. Lyme disease is caused by *B. burgdorferi* via the Ixodes deer tick. Lyme presents in multiple stages, spreading from local to multisystem:

Stage 1 (early): Erythema migrans (targetoid lesion)

Stage 2: Third-degree AV block, facial nerve palsy (Bell's), migratory arthritis, and myalgias

Stage 3 (late): Encephalopathy and chronic arthritis

Typically patients on the shelf will present with either stage 1 or 2 symptoms, although be wary of stage 3 when considering the differential for encephalopathies. Also keep a keen eye out for exposure to tall grass and hiking in the Northeastern US.

Be sure to differentiate Lyme from *Babesia microti*, which is also transmitted by Ixodes tick but will present with hemolytic anemia instead (Fig. 3.1).

PPx: (1) Avoid skin exposure while hiking in tall grass in the Northeastern US.

MoD: Ixodes deer tick → *B. burgdorferi* bacterium transmitted through bite to patient → Lyme disease

Dx:

1. Complete blood count (CBC), basic metabolic panel (BMP)
2. ELISA, confirm w/ WB

Tx/Mgmt:

1. If older than 9 years old: doxycycline; in kids younger than 9 years, treat with amoxicillin

Lyme disease patient presentation

2. If disseminated (e.g., stage 3), ceftriaxone if doxycycline not an answer choice

Q Fever (Coxiella burnetii)

Buzz Words: Exposure to cattle or sheep + pneumonia + endocarditis (culture negative) + no rash → Q fever 2/2 *C. burnetii*

Clinical Presentation: Most common chief complaint is pneumonia, but for the family medicine shelf, keep this on your radar in patients with culture negative endocarditis. Rarely tested. Be sure to know Buzz Words to identify disease in question stem.

PPx: (1) Avoidance of cattle or sheep

MoD: *C. burnetii* bacteria transmitted through spores from cattle or sheep secretions

Dx, Tx/Mgmt: Do not need to know for Family Medicine shelf

Rickettsiosis (Rocky Mountain Spotted Fever)

Buzz Words: Headache + fever + rash that starts in the wrist and spreads proximally/distally + rash of palms and soles + pancytopenia + hyponatremia → Rocky Mountain Spotted Fever (RMSF)

Clinical Presentation: RMSF is a disease commonly seen on the East Coast. The rash starts at the wrist and spreads to the palms and soles. Do not look for "went hiking in the Rocky Mountains" in the question stem as that is NOT a buzz word (too obvious and patients are typically not from the Rocky Mountain region). Patients are treated with doxycycline. Make sure to know the differential of diseases that present with rash in the palms and soles (RMSF, syphilis, and hand-foot-mouth disease) as it is a buzz word that helps you easily distinguish disease.

PPx: (1) Avoidance of hiking in the East Coast

MoD: (1) Rickettsia is carried by and transmitted through the dermacentor tick

Dx:

1. Clinical

Tx/Mgmt:

1. Doxycycline (no age restriction)

> **QUICK TIPS**
> Rash of the palms or soles of foot → only three diseases should be on your differential; Hand-foot-mouth disease caused by coxsackie A virus (pretty obvious), syphilis (secondary), and RMSF.

Infectious Mononucleosis (aka "Mono")

Buzz Words: Young adult + posterior cervical lymphadenopathy + fever/fatigue + hepatosplenomegaly + exudative pharyngitis + cold autoimmune hemolytic anemia (e.g., painful extremities w/ hemolytic anemia) + heterophile antibodies → infectious mononucleosis

Young adult + persistent abdominal pain after trauma (e.g., physical contact during sports) to left upper quadrant + shock + recent history of fever/sickness that had "resolved" → rupture of the spleen 2/2 hepatospleno-megaly from mononucleosis infection

Fever/fatigue + polymorphous maculopapular rash s/p amoxicillin → Indicative of infection with Epstein-Barr virus (EBV) (rash seems to occur when amoxicillin is given in s/o EBV infection; not considered a drug allergy and mechanism unknown)

Burkitt's lymphoma + nasopharyngeal carcinoma → EBV infection

Tonsillar exudates + fever + anterior lymphadenopathy → GA strep pharyngitis (vs. mono which has posterior LAD; Fig. 3.2)

Fever + fatigue + exudative pharyngitis + tonsillar exudates + diffuse, posterior cervical LAD + splenomegaly (and hepatomegaly) → infectious mononucleosis

Clinical Presentation: Mono is the most high-yield multisystem viral infection because it is commonly seen, affects many different organ systems (e.g., upper respiratory tract, liver, spleen). Furthermore, EBV, the infectious agent, has been implicated in a couple of well-known cancers (e.g., Burkitt's lymphoma and nasopharyngeal carcinoma).

PPx: (1) Avoid kissing someone with mono (or anyone with a fever/is clearly sick); (2) if infected, avoid sports for at least three weeks to prevent splenic rupture.

QUICK TIPS

Complications of EBV-mediated mono: (1) increased risk for splenic rupture, (2) rash if exposed to PCN, (3) can remain dormant in B cells → increases risk of recurrence and lymphoma (pathoma)

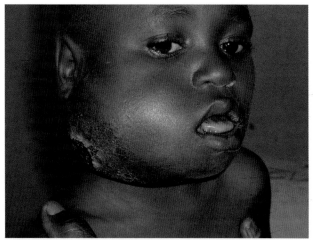

FIG. 3.2 Burkitt's lymphoma jaw swelling. Wikipedia: https://en.wikipedia.org/wiki/Burkitt%27s_lymphoma#/media/File:Large_facial_Burkitt%27s_Lymphoma.JPG

MoD: Caused by EBV (aka HHV-4) transmitted through saliva ("kissing") → infects B cells through CD21

Dx:
1. Monospot
2. Positive heterophile antibody test (will show antibodies detected by agglutination of animal red blood cells)

Tx/Mgmt:
1. Supportive care
2. Steroids

Cytomegalovirus Infection

Buzz Words: Healthy adult + posterior lymphadenopathy + hepatosplenomegaly + sore throat + monospot **negative** → CMV infection in the immunocompetent

HIV + mucosal inflammation + epithelial cells w/ large ovoid nuclei + prominent basophilic deposits + **retinal detachment**

IV drug user + previous pneumocystis dx + white/opaque patches at retinal periphery

Owl eye inclusion in mononuclear cells + cotton-wool exudates and hemorrhage

Clinical Presentation: Cytomegalovirus infections should be thought of on a spectrum according to the strength of a patient's immune system. Healthy adults who are infected by cytomegalovirus (CMV) through bodily fluids (e.g., saliva, sexual contact) experience a mononucleosis-like syndrome (e.g., posterior LAD, pharyngitis) but is Monospot negative (i.e., mono not mediated by EBV). Those who are immunocompromised, however, experience much graver consequences, including vision loss 2/2 retinitis in s/o AIDS, pneumonia (particularly in kidney transplant patients), encephalitis, and esophagitis and ulceration of gastrointestinal (GI) tract in AIDS patients.

Be mindful that CMV will present completely differently in the pediatric population (e.g., peds shelf). It is one of the ToRCHeS infections that can transfer directly from mother to baby. Congenital CMV presents classically with periventricular calcifications, seizures, rash, and hearing loss; however you will likely only see this presentation on your Peds shelf.

PPx: (1) Use condoms; (2) reduce morbidity of disease through immunocompetence (e.g., tx/ppx of AIDS); (3) if pregnant, treat mom to avoid congenital CMV.

MoD: Transmission through bodily fluids, such as saliva, sexual contact, urine, blood

FOR THE WARDS

Monospot test detects IgM antibodies that cross-react with horse or sheep RBCs (heterophile antibodies). Positive monospot = agglutination occurs = EBV infection. Negative monospot = no agglutination = CMV infection

Dx:
1. Monospot (will be **negative**, meaning no agglutination)
2. If immunocompromised, fundoscopic exam
3. Endoscopy (may show ulceration of GI tract)
4. Biopsy of ulceration → intranuclear inclusions

Tx/Mgmt:
1. Ganciclovir (may lead to agranulocytosis)
2. Foscarnet for AIDS retinitis
3. Cidofovir if refractory to treatment

Fungal Infections

These fungal infections are very high yield for the shelf. For blastomycosis, coccidioidomycosis and histoplasma, in particular, you will be asked to identify disease based on the geographic region of travel. Make sure to know the buzz words and clinical presentations of these fungal infections very well. Mechanism of disease and diagnostic steps (e.g., what these yeast look like on biopsy and culture) are topics for step 1 and not the shelf exam; they are included here to for completeness sake but can be skipped over if you are pressed for time.

Candidiasis (*Candida albicans*)

Buzz Words: Thick, white curd-like, discharge, itching, satellite lesions + no odor + KOH positive → vaginal candidiasis

Thick, white plaques in oral mucosa + KOH positive → oral thrush

Erythematous, eroded patches w/ satellite lesions + KOH positive → cutaneous candidiasis

Clinical Presentation: Candidiasis is a mucocutaneous infection in which candida species (most commonly *albicans*) grows in damp environments, such as oral mucosa, skin folds, and genitalia. Can be associated with immunocompromised states if found in certain parts of the body (e.g., *Candida* in oropharynx). Definitive diagnosis is with KOH wet mount and treatment is with antifungals.

PPx: (1) Risk factors such as DM, abx use, immunosuppression, HIV/AIDS

MoD: Candida resides harmlessly on dry skin → begins to grow in damp, hot environments with impaired immune defenses

Dx:
1. Clinical
2. KOH prep (budding yeast + pseudohyphae)

Tx/Mgmt:
1. Fluconazole or miconazole cream (vaginal)
2. Nystatin powder (cutaneous)
3. Nystatin "swish and-swallow" (thrush)

Parasitic

This section is largely a holdover from step 1 material. Make sure to know the buzz words and how to distinguish the clinical presentation of one parasitic infection from another. PPx, MoD, Dx and Tx/Mgmt won't be tested on the shelf.

TABLE 3.2 Comparison of Blastomycosis, Coccidioidomycosis, and Histoplasmosis (Further Covered in Chapter 8)

	Blastomycosis	Coccidioidomycosis (aka San Joaquin Fever)	Histoplasmosis
Buzz Words	• Pneumonia • granulomas in skin and bone • Central America/Great Lakes/East Coast	• Mild respiratory sx → PNA • granulomas in skin (erythema nodosum) and musculoskeletal (arthralgia) • s/p earthquakes • SW US or Central/South America	• Pneumonia Mississippi/Ohio River valleys • Cave (e.g., contact with bats) • Hiking (e.g., contact with birds)
Clinical Presentation (all three can form **granulomas**)	Blastomycosis is an inflammatory lung disease that can dis-seminate to skin and bone. Geographically, patients are either from the Great Lakes, the East Coast of the United States, or Central America.	Coccidioidomycosis is usually asymptom-atic, but patients can present with mild respiratory symptoms and concomitant skin and bone involvement. Infection can occur after earthquakes that shake up fungal spores. Geographically, patients are from SW US, San Joaquin Valley, South America.	Histoplasmosis is usu-ally asymptomatic but can present with mild respiratory symptoms or pneumonia. Disease associated with contact with bats (e.g., caves) and birds (e.g., hiking). Geographically, patients are from Mississippi and Ohio River valleys.
PPx (no human transmission)	(1) Avoid endemic areas	(1) Avoid endemic areas	(1) avoid endemic areas
MoD	*Blastomyces dermatitidis*	*Coccidioides immitis/ posadasii*	*Histoplasma capsulatum*

Continued

TABLE 3.2 Comparison of Blastomycosis, Coccidioidomycosis, and Histoplasmosis (Further Covered in Chapter 8)—cont'd

	Blastomycosis	Coccidioidomycosis (aka San Joaquin Fever)	Histoplasmosis
Dx **Do not need to know in detail for the shelf exam** (however, important for step 1)	• Biopsy shows single broad-based bud -Thick-walled budding yeast at 37°C + hyphae w/ small conidia at 25°C • Dimorphic systemic fungi (e.g., mold outside body but yeast within body)	Biopsy shows huge **spherule** w/ endospores • Fungal endospores w/ spherules at 37°C + branched hyphae at 25°C • Only fungi that is not dimorphic because exists as spherule	Biopsy shows macrophage-filled spores seen **within the macrophage** • Dimorphic systemic fungi
Tx/Mgmt	(1) Itraconazole (or another –azole such as ketoconazole), (2) amphotericin B	(1) Itraconazole, (2) amphotericin b	(1) Itraconazole, (2) amphotericin B

Schistosomiasis (Schistosoma)

Buzz Words: Hepatosplenomegaly + hematuria + granulomatous pulmonary disease + portal hypertension + exposure to snails

Clinical Presentation: Can present with dystrophic calcification, granulomas, and portal hypertension. Infectious agent is a trematode (worm). Patient in the question stem may present with hepatosplenomegaly or hematuria (squamous cell carcinoma of the bladder). May have an exposure to snails. While common for step 1, uncommon on the shelf exam.

PPx, MoD, Dx, Tx/Mgmt: Not tested on the shelf

Leishmaniasis (*Leishmania* spp.), Visceral (Kalaazar)

Buzz Words: Fever + pancytopenia + hepatosplenomegaly + ulcers + recent travel to South America (e.g., exposure to sandfly)

Clinical Presentation: Leishmaniasis is a protozoal infection mediated by the sandfly that is tested mostly on step 1 and not on the shelf. It can be distinguished from other parasitic infections by its combination of pancytopenia and fevers. Know only the buzz words for this disease.

PPx, MoD, Dx, Tx/Mgmt: Not tested on the shelf

Trypanosomiasis/Chagas Disease, Acute and Chronic (Trypanosoma)

Buzz Words: South America + dilated cardiomyopathy + hypertrophy of the GI tract (e.g., esophagus, colon) + periorbital swelling

Clinical Presentation: Patients with Chagas disease classically have come home from a recent trip to a South American country (e.g., Brazil, Chile) and have pain and swelling of one eye (acute) and later may present with expansion for cardiologic and GI structures (e.g., dilated ventricles, hypertrophied esophagus/colon). Transmission is through the reduviid bug from a painless bite. Like the other systemic parasites, Chagas disease is more step 1 than shelf. Feel free to skip if pressed for time.

PPx, MoD, Dx, Tx/Mgmt: Not tested on the shelf

Autoimmune Disorders

Autoimmune disorders are characterized by damaged tissues from aberrant attacks from one's own immune system. These typically affect multiple organ systems and thus are high yield on the Family Medicine shelf. In addition, many of these autoimmune disorders, such as systemic lupus erythematosus (SLE), are known as great imitators and should be on the differential for most chief complaints.

Systemic Lupus Erythematosus (aka Lupus)

Buzz Words: RPR and VDRL positive + elevated PTT + recurrent abortions + malar rash → antiphospholipid antibody in s/o SLE

Can be primary d/o or associated with SLE.

Antihistone antibody + malar rash + new drug/medication → drug-induced lupus

IgG + Malar rash + Discoid rash + ANA + Mucositis (mouth ulcers) + Neuro dysfunction + Serositis (pleuritis/pericarditis) + Hematologic d/o (pancytopenia) + arthritis + Renal d/o (wire loops) + Photosensitivity + Psychosis → SLE

Clinical Presentation: SLE is an autoimmune disorder that can present as nearly any chief complaint and is thus often kept somewhere on the differential. It is thus very easy to get lost when thinking about SLE. Here are two organizing principles to guide your study.

QUICK TIPS
Antiphospholipid antibodies include (1) lupus anticoagulant (elevates PTT), (2) anticardiolipin (false positive VDRL and RPR), (3) anti-beta 2-glycoprotein

QUICK TIPS
Antiphospholipid d/o characterized by hypercoagulable state 2/2 antiphospholipid antibodies

QUICK TIPS
Agents (e.g., slow acetylators in the liver) that lead to drug-induced lupus: SLE caused by sulfa HIPP-E's (sulfa drugs, Hydralazine, Isoniazid, Procainamide, Phenytoin, Etanercept)

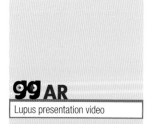

First, be clear on how SLE presents on the shelf. Although, SLE is the "great imitator," there are only a handful of Buzz Words or clinical vignettes that can be used to describe SLE. First, be on the lookout for a (most likely) female patient with a malar (e.g., "butterfly") rash over the bridge of her nose who presents with constitutional symptoms, such as fatigue, fever, and night sweats (Fig. 3.3).

On the shelf, these patients typically have been recently exposed to sun (e.g., beach trip) or perhaps forgot to put on sunscreen. In addition, the shelf may try to trick you by showing either (a) lab results that falsely suggest syphilis (e.g., VDRL and RPR positive) or (b) lab results that falsely suggest a hematologic disorder (e.g., elevated PTT). Be very suspicious that these findings are due to antiphospholipid antibodies (e.g., lupus anticoagulant). For the Family Medicine shelf, these findings may present as a woman with a history of recurrent spontaneous abortions, a sequelae of having circulating lupus anticoagulant. In addition, anytime someone is positive anti-dsDNA or anti-Sm antibodies, know that is pathognomonic for SLE. SLE patients are also ANA positive, but ANA is not specific for the disease. Finally, patients with anti-histone antibodies have drug-induced

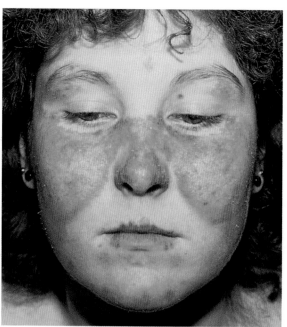

FIG. 3.3 Malar rash. (From Katarzyna Gilek-Seibert: Systemic lupus erythematosus. In Ferri F, *Ferri's Clinical Advisor*. Elsevier; 2018.)

lupus. Knowing these aforementioned Buzz Words will help you avoid confusion and immediately sniff out what the NBME examiners are up to.

Second, for your clerkship rotation, remember that SLE can affect every organ system due to deposition of immune complexes. Make sure you have a systematic way to think through how the disease may present, such as telling a story from head to toe (e.g., face/sun-exposed skin → malar or discoid rash, photosensitive; brain → seizures, psychosis; respiratory tract → inflammation of lung pleura; heart → pericarditis, Libman-Sacks endocarditis; GI tract → oropharyngeal ulcers; genitourinary tract (including kidneys) → diffuse proliferative glomerulonephritis with deposits on the subendothelium, membranous glomerulonephritis with deposits on the subepithelium, kidney failure; musculoskeletal → inflammatory arthritis (usually at least two joints); hematologic → leukopenia (more susceptible to infection), anemia, thrombocytopenia, hypercoagulant (more susceptible to CAD, thrombosis in placenta during pregnancy); male/female reproductive system → mucositis, recurrent pregnancy loss secondary to thrombosis; endocrine → thyroid autoimmunity. Lastly, remember that most SLE patients die from renal failure (most commonly from DPGN), so keep a keen eye on renal function and be prepared to counsel patients accordingly.

PPx: (1) Sunscreen (avoid sun exposure)

MoD:

1. Mostly considered type 3 hypersensitivity because damage is mediated by antigen-antibody immune complexes

   Sun damage → apoptotic debris → activation and production of antibodies that target antigens from patient cell nucleus → immune complex formed → immune complex deposited in body tissues and upregulates immune responses (using up complement proteins leading to deficient C1, C2, and C4)

2. In pregnancy, Lupus anticoagulant leads to thrombus development within the placenta → spontaneous abortion/pregnancy loss

3. Pancytopenia in SLE mediated by direct antibody attack on RBCs, WBCs and platelets (type 2 hypersensitivity)

Dx:

1. CBC/BMP
2. ANA

99 AR

Libman-Sacks endocarditis a form of nonbacterial endocarditis mediated by vegetations and associated with SLE

99 AR

Thyroid autoimmunity associated with SLE

QUICK TIPS

PTT is artificially elevated in lupus. RPR and VDRL are falsely positive in lupus as well.

3. Anti-Smith and anti-dsDNA antibodies (specific/golden standard for diagnosis)
4. Complement levels (may show decrease C1, C3, C4)

Tx/Mgmt:
1. Nonsteroidal anti-inflammatory drugs (NSAIDs)
2. Steroids
3. Anticoagulation (e.g., warfarin, heparin) if antiphospho-lipid antibody syndrome
4. D/c drug if drug-induced lupus
5. DMARDs (e.g., Methotrexate)
6. Biologics (e.g., TNF alpha inhibitors), v2. renal transplant if kidney failure

Lupus Treatment in Pregnancy

- NSAIDs only for arthralgia/serositis and NOT for acute flares
- Steroids for acute flares
- Hydroxychloroquine → control skin manifestations; may cause lupus flare if d/c'd

Sjogren Syndrome

Buzz Words: Enlarged parotid glands (like a chipmunk) + dry eyes + dry mouth + anti-Ro (SSA) and anti-La (SSB) antibodies → Sjogren syndrome

Sjogren + joint pain → Sjogren with concomitant rheumatoid arthritis

Clinical Presentation: Sjogren syndrome is an autoimmune disorder characterized by lymphocytic damage to salivary and lacrimal glands. Patients are usually older women who present with enlarged parotid glands, dry mouth (perhaps as recurrent dental infections), and dry eyes. Like many autoimmune disorders, Sjogren syndrome can be associated with other autoimmune pathology. Folks with Sjogren syndrome often present with rheumatoid arthritis, SLE, systemic sclerosis, or primary biliary cirrhosis. Diagnosis is made by anti-SSA or anti-SSB antibodies, although a biopsy of the salivary/lacrimal glands can also be used to confirm. Complications of Sjogren syndrome include marginal zone lymphoma and acute interstitial nephritis.

PPx: None

MoD: Damage in Sjogren syndrome is mediated by lymphocytes and is therefore considered a type 4 hypersensitivity reaction. Lymphocytes attack lacrimal and salivary glands → dry mouth and dry eyes → dental infections and eyes susceptible to abrasion.

Dx:
1. CBC/BMP
2. ANA (positive)
3. Rheumatoid factor (r/o rheumatoid arthritis, which is often concomitant)
4. Anti-SSA (anti-ro) and anti-SSB (anti-La) antibodies
5. Biopsy of salivary glands (shows lymphocytic infiltration)

Tx/Mgmt:
1. Eye drops for dry eyes
2. Pilocarpine for dry mouth
3. Corticosteroids

Systemic Sclerosis (aka Scleroderma)

Buzz Words: Anti-scl-70 + tightening of skin all over body + gastroesophageal reflux disease (GERD) + Raynauds + pulmonary hypertension → scleroderma (diffuse)

Anti-centromere antibody + sclerodactyly + tightening of skin on hand/face only + Raynaud phenomenon + esophageal dysmotility + telangiectasias + calcinosis → scleroderma (limited, aka CREST syndrome; Fig. 3.4)

Clinical Presentation: Scleroderma is an autoimmune disorder that is characterized by fibrosis of skin and internal organs. Like other autoimmune disorders, it more commonly is seen in females (middle aged). It is divided into two types of disease: diffuse and limited. Diffuse scleroderma means the fibrosis characteristic of the disease can occur anywhere in the body, and frequently leads to death through pulmonary hypertension. Limited scleroderma is known as CREST syndrome due to the mnemonic: Calcinosis/antiCentromere antibody; Raynaud phenomenon; Esophageal dysmotility; Sclerodactyly; Telangiectasia. For the shelf, the easiest way to distinguish the two entities is through the presence of antibodies: Anti-scl-70 = diffuse scleroderma; anti-centromere = limited scleroderma. Unlike SLE and Sjogren syndrome, you will only mainly be responsible for identifying this disease in the clinical presentation rather than knowing the diagnostic and treatment steps.

PPx: None

MoD: Endothelial damage → inflammation and increased growth factors → fibrosis + deposition of collagen on organs (exact etiology still unknown)

Dx:
1. CBC/BMP
2. Anti-scl-70 and anti-centromere antibody

FOR THE WARDS

Raynaud Phenomenon: When arterioles of distal extremities vasospasm 2/2 cold exposure → white/blue hands and feet. Treatment is to keep distal extremities warm (e.g., move to warm climate, gloves) and CCBs.

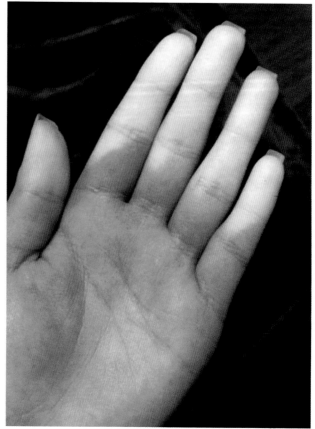

FIG. 3.4 Raynaud phenomenon.

Tx/Mgmt:
1. Supportive according to symptom (e.g., gloves/warm weather for patients with Raynaud phenomenon, PPI for patients with GERD)

Mixed Connective Tissue Disease

Buzz Words: Anti-U1 ribonucleoprotein antibodies + ANA + features of SLE, scleroderma, and polymyositis

Clinical Presentation: Mixed connective tissue disease (MCTD) is an autoimmune disorder that combines features of three prominent autoimmune disorders (e.g., polymyositis, SLE, and scleroderma). On the shelf, the only thing you will be tested on is disease recognition or the ability to eliminate this as an answer choice. Recognize that anti-U1 ribonucleoprotein antibodies are associated with MCTD and move on.

Reactive Arthritis (aka Reiter Disease/ Reiter Arthritis)

Buzz Words: Conjunctivitis + urethral discharge + arthralgia + pericarditis/aortic regurg + history of STIs or GI infection + HLA B27 → Reactive arthritis

Clinical Presentation: Reactive arthritis is one of the seronegative spondyloarthropathies, which means an arthritis that does not have an anti-IgG antibody (non-rheumatoid). It is associated with HLA-B27, and has a classic triad of conjunctivitis, urethritis, and arthritis (can't see, can't pee, can't climb up a tree). Know how to identify reactive arthritis on the shelf, and keep a keen eye out for antecedent infections, such chlamydia (STI) and bacterial GI infections (campylobacter, shigella, salmonella).

PPx: (1) Avoid chlamydia and GI infections

MoD: Unknown, but can be triggered by an STI (*Chlamydia trachomatis*) or a GI infection (*Campylobacter jejuni*, *Salmonella*, or *Shigella*)

Dx:
1. CBC/BMP
2. XR of affected arthritic joints
3. Fundoscopic exam for conjunctivitis
4. UA/UCx for urethritis
5. Genetic testing for HLA-B27

Tx/Mgmt:
1. Antibiotics
2. Steroids
3. Symptom specific

Sexually Transmitted Infections

Screening guidelines for STIs are particularly important for the Family Medicine exam. The full list can be found on the Centers for Disease Control and Prevention (CDC) website (link in the Gunner Column). However, be careful not to get bogged down in all the details. Instead, focus on learning the screening guidelines that are most commonly tested. These are included in the PPx section.

Bacterial Vaginosis

Buzz words: White-to-gray thin discharge + fishy odor + clue cells + pH >4.5, positive whiff test

Clinical Presentation: Bacterial vaginosis (BV) is an overgrowth of normal vaginal bacteria, and is the most common cause of vaginitis. It's not an STD, as it's not caused by infection by foreign bacteria. There is not one single type of bacteria that causes BV, as it can be caused by the overgrowth of various normal vaginal bacteria. However, it can cause frustrating symptoms to the patient. Some patients are prone to getting BV frequently, whereas others rarely do. The imbalance in normal flora causes white-gray vaginal discharge, notable odor, and the odor gets worse after sex. On exam, the vaginal pH, which is normally around 4, will increase to over 4.5 (alkaline), and you will see clue cells on a wet mount slide under the microscope, which are epithelial cells covered in dots of bacteria. Adding potassium hydroxide (KOH) to a sample of the vaginal discharge on a microscope will cause a very fishy odor; this is called a positive Whiff Test. Risk factors include having sex (though patients can get BV without having sex) and vaginal douching.

PPx: (1) Avoid vaginal douching, which alters normal flora

MoD: Overgrowth of normal vaginal bacteria

Dx:

1. Vaginal discharge with a pH >4.5
2. Clue cells under the microscope
3. Positive Whiff Test: very fishy odor when adding KOH to sample of discharge

Tx/Mgmt:

1. Metronidazole or Clindamycin, can be given orally or vaginally. Treatment is indicated for pregnant women with BV, as untreated BV during pregnancy can cause preterm birth. Warn your patient to not drink alcohol while taking metronidazole as this can cause disulfram-like reaction.

99 AR

Clue cells under the microscope: epithelial cells covered in "dots" of bacteria

Trichomonas

Buzz Words: Gray/yellow/green discharge + strawberry cervix + pH >4.5 + corkscrew motility

Clinical Presentation: *Trichomonas vaginalis* is a sexually transmitted flagellated protozoa that causes vaginitis in women. Symptomatic women present with vaginal itching or burning and a frothy, grey, yellow, or green vaginal discharge with a musty or fishy odor (although the KOH Whiff Test is sometimes positive with trichomoniasis, remember that "fishy odor" and a positive Whiff Test on exams is the buzzword for BV). Women may also have an inflamed cervix with red petechia on pelvic exam, classically called "strawberry cervix." Men and women are both affected; however, men rarely have symptoms, and up to half of all women who are affected do not have symptoms either. The pH of the vaginal discharge is greater than 4.5, and under the microscope you will see the flagellated protozoa "swimming" across the slide, sometimes called "corkscrew" or "quivering" motility. Because *T. vaginalis* is an STI, patients with multiple sexual partners who do not use a condom are at the highest risk.

PPx: (1) Counsel on condom use, (2) treat partner with metronidazole

MoD: This flagellated protozoa is transmitted sexually most often from male to female during sex, but can be transmitted from female to male and female to female.

Dx:

1. Visualization of protozoa under microscope

Tx/Mgmt:

1. Metronidazole or Tindazole. Can treat during pregnancy, as untreated *T. vaginalis* is associated with premature birth and low birth weight. Warn patients not to drink alcohol with either of these medications as it may cause disulfram-like reaction.

99 AR

Protozoa with flagella on wet mount

99 AR

Strawberry cervix on pelvic exam

Urinary Tract Infection (Cystitis)

Buzz Words: Honeymoon + catheter + dysuria (burning on urination) + frequency + urgency, suprapubic tenderness, occasional fever

Clinical Presentation: Urinary tract infections (UTIs) are much more prevalent in women than in men. Risk factors include pregnancy, indwelling catheters, diabetes (increases the risk of ascension to kidneys) and structural abnormality.

PPx: Bladder infection

MoD: Usually ascending infection from the urethra

Escherichia coli — most common cause

Staphylococcus saprophyticus — sexually active young woman

Enterococcus, Klebsielle, Proteus, Pseudomonas, Enterobacter — catheter

Dx:

1. Urine dipstick
2. Leukocyte esterase — indicates white blood cells in urine (pyuria)
3. Nitrite — positive for gram-negative bacteria. *Negative nitrite does not exclude cystitis*

Tx/Mgmt:

1. Asymptomatic—two successive positive cultures with >10^5 CFUs (treated only if patient is pregnant or going to have urologic surgery)
2. Uncomplicated (empiric treatment is appropriate): Oral **TMP/SMX** is first line, and Nitrofurantoin or fosfomycin or fluoroquinolones is second line

Chlamydia

Buzz Words: <24 years + purulent discharge + dysuria + gram negative

Clinical Presentation: Presents as purulent discharge, abnormal bleeding, dysuria. Chlamydia is the most common bacterial STD and is often asymptomatic. It is a risk factor for cancer and is a leading cause of infertility 2/2 scarring.

PPx: (1) Screen all sexually active women younger than 25 years, (2) screen sexually active women older than 25 years if at high risk (e.g., past history of STIs), (3) screen men at high risk (e.g., history of STIs, MSM), (4) screen all pregnant women younger than 25 years during third trimester, (5) counsel on protective barriers during sex (condoms).

MoD: Intracellular pathogen

Dx:

1. Nucleic acid amplification test (NAAT)
2. Gram stain (should be negative)

Tx/Mgmt:

1. Azithromycin or doxycycline
2. Retest 3 months after treatment

Gonorrhea

Buzz Words: Migratory polyarthritis + endocarditis + rash

Clinical Presentation: Gonorrhea is one of the most common STDs and can cause cervicitis, PID, tubulovarian abscess, Fitz-Hugh-Curtis and infertility in females. In males, gonorrhea can present as epididymitis.

PPx: (1) Screen all sexually active women older than 25 years, (2) screen sexually active women younger than 25 years if at high risk (e.g., past history of STIs), (3) screen men at high risk (e.g., history of STIs, MSM), (4) screen all pregnant women younger than 25 years during third trimester, (5) counsel on protective barriers during sex (condoms).

MoD: Sexual transmission

Dx:
1. Nucleic acid amplification test (NAAT)
2. Gram stain (should be positive)

Tx/Mgmt:
1. Ceftriaxone + azithromycin (assumes concomitant chlamydia infection)
2. Hospitalization if disseminated

Pelvic Inflammatory Disease

Buzz Words: Cervical motion tenderness + chandelier sign

Clinical Presentation: Pelvic inflammatory disease (PID) occurs when an infection of the vagina ascends to the cervix, uterus, fallopian tubes, ovaries, or beyond. The most common causes are *Neisseria gonorrhea* and *Chlamydia trachomatis*. It's not uncommon for more than one bacterial culprit. Women often complain of low abdominal pain, cramps, fever, and cervical motion tenderness on exam. Patients often has so much pain that they "jump to the chandelier" when performing a pelvic exam and feeling the patient's cervix, known as the Chandelier Sign. Patients also can have adnexal tenderness. Because PID is often a sequela of untreated STIs, risk factors include having multiple sexual partners and not using a condom. Complications of untreated PID include adhesions causing infertility.

PPx: (1) Use condom (2) treat STI before progression to PID

MoD: STI with bacteria such as *Neisseria gonorrhea* or *Chlamydia trachomatis* ascends female reproductive tract into uterus, fallopian tubes, ovaries, or further into pelvis.

Dx:
1. Clinical diagnosis with constellation of symptoms and cervical motion tenderness or adnexal tenderness
2. Laparoscopy (definitive diagnosis)

Tx/Mgmt:
1. Treatment is Ceftriaxone or Cefoxitin or Cefotetan plus Doxycycline, or Clindamycin plus Gentamycin.

> **QUICK TIPS**
>
> Patients with suspected PID on clinical exam should be treated with antibiotics due to the risk of infertility, tubo-ovarian abscess, or Fitz-Hugh-Curtis syndrome with untreated PID.

Chancroid

Buzz Words: Painful chancre + inguinal lymphadenopathy, school of fish on Gram stain

Clinical Presentation: Painful genital area 2–10 days after sexual contact

PPx: Condoms

MoD: Sexual transmission

Dx:
1. Must rule out syphilis, HSV

Tx/Mgmt: Azithromycin, ceftriaxone, erythromycin, ciprofloxacin; resolution within 1–2 weeks

Genital Herpes

Buzz Words: Painful + vesicular → herpes, Bell's palsy

Clinical Presentation: Painful recurrent oral and genital vesicles with the potential to rupture. Dissemination may occur, especially in pregnant women and the immunocompromised. Patients have increased risk of catching HIV:

- HSV-1 typically on oropharynx, though can infect genitals (associated with Bell's palsy)
- HSV-2 typically on genitals, though can infect oropharynx

PPx: (1) Consider screening in high-risk patients (e.g., multiple sex partners, MSM, HIV, history of STIs); however, not mandatory, (2) counsel on condom use

MoD: Replication in dermis/epidermis before retrograde travel to dorsal root ganglia

Dx: Usually clinically.
1. **Tzanck** is quickest (uses Wright stain)
2. Culture is gold standard

Tx/Mgmt
1. Acyclovir, valacyclovir, foscarnet

Human Papillomavirus

Buzz Words: Genital wart, cervical dysplasia, cancer

Clinical Presentation: One of the most common STDs. Has multiple strains. HPV6-11 is low risk and leads to condyloma acuminatum (genital warts). HPV 16–18, 31, 33, 45 are high-risk strains that can lead to cervical dysplasia and cancer.

PPx: (1) Gardasil: quadrivalent vaccine indicated for women 11–26 years old and men 11–21 years old. (2) Screen women 21–29 years of age every 3 years with cytology. (3) Screen women 30–65 years old every 3 years with cytology OR every 5 years with cytology + HPV. (4) Frequency of screening increased for women with HIV (within 1 year of sexual activity or initial HIV diagnosis, then repeat testing 6 months afterward).

MoD: Skin-skin contact

Dx:
1. Clinical

Tx/Mgmt:
1. Podophyllin
2. Cryotherapy or laser for genital warts

Lymphogranuloma Venereum

Buzz Words: painless ulcers + small, shallow ulcers + matted lymph nodes + buboes + sinus tracts
Clinical Presentation: Has three stages: Primary = transient and painless ulcer, secondary = painful lymphadenopathy, tertiary = anogenital syndrome (proctocolitis, rectal strictures, rectovaginal fistula)
PPx: (1) Condoms
MoD: (1) Caused by *Chlamydia trachomatis* serovars L1–3 (different from the serotypes that cause chlamydia vaginitis/urethritis)
Dx:
1. Clinical
2. ELISA to look for antibodies to chlamydia endotoxin
Tx/Mgmt:
1. Doxycycline
2. Erythromycin
3. Drainage of buboes

Syphilis

Buzz Words: Painless ulcer + lymphadenopathy + treponemes on dark field microscopy → Primary syphilis
Rash of palms and soles + condyloma lata + general lymphadenopathy → secondary syphilis
Argyll Robertson pupils + gummas + neurosyphilis + aortitis → tertiary syphilis
Clinical Presentation: Syphilis is one of the great imitators and should always be on the differential for any chief complaint. For the shelf, make sure to know both the **congenital** and the **adult** (see above) presentations of the disease.
PPx: (1) Screen all pregnant women at first prenatal visit and third semester, (2) annual screen for men who have sex with men (MSM), (3) annual screen for patients with HIV, (4) counsel on condoms.
MoD: (1) Caused by the spirochete *Treponema pallidum*
Dx:
1. RPR
2. VDRL
3. Fluorescent treponemal antibody absorption test (FTA)

QUICK TIPS
Argyll Robertson pupil = prostitute's pupil (i.e., accommodates but does not react)

QUICK TIPS
Congenital syphilis (e.g., vertical transmission from mom to newborn) presents differently and has different buzz words depending on younger or older than 2 years of age.

QUICK TIPS

VDRL false positives include **lupus (or lupus anticoagulant)**, rheumatic fever, drugs, and viral infection

4. Dark-field microscopy (definitive diagnosis)
5. HIV and HBV

Tx/Mgmt:

1. Penicillin
2. If allergic to penicillin, desensitize by incremental doses of PO penicillin

GUNNER PRACTICE

1. A 33-year-old man comes to the physician 2 days after an itchy rash developed on his hands, forearms, arms, and face. He reports returning from a recent camping trip and states how happy he was that he protected himself with ample sunscreen, a wide-brimmed hat, and copious amounts of bug spray. He recalls being adventurous and wading through "many bushes and leaves." His vital signs are within normal limits. On exam, there is a linear pattern of red papules and vesicles on his arms and face. Otherwise, no abnormalities are found. What is the mechanism for the rash seen on this patient?
   A. Hypersensitivity, type 1
   B. Hypersensitivity, type 2
   C. Hypersensitivity, type 3
   D. Hypersensitivity, type 4
   E. Jarisch-Herxheimer reaction

2. A 29-year-old female with a history of HIV for 5 years comes to the physician for a follow-up appointment. She is compliant with her medication and has no trouble controlling her symptoms. She is currently taking the HAART regimen and a proton pump inhibitor for GERD. Her last CD4 count was 545 cells/cubic millimeter. She does, however, endorse being around people who cough all the time recently, from her significant other to her parents who live nearby. What is the next most appropriate step?
   A. Reassurance
   B. Prescribe anxiolytic
   C. PPD skin test
   D. Spirometry
   E. Chest X-ray

Notes

ANSWERS: What Would Gunner Jess/Jim Do?

1. WWGJD? A 33-year-old man comes to the physician 2 days after an itchy rash developed on his hands, forearms, arms and face. He reports returning from a recent camping trip and states how happy he was that he protected himself with ample sunscreen, a wide-brimmed hat, and copious amounts of bug spray. He recalls being adventurous and **wading through "many bushes and leaves."** His vital signs are within normal limits. On exam, there is a **linear pattern of red papules and vesicles on his arms and face.** Otherwise, no abnormalities are found. What is the mechanism for the rash seen on this patient?

   Answer: D, Hypersensitivity, type 4

      Explanation: Given the patient's history, it is likely that he got poison ivy or poison oak from forays into nature. What gives it away are the clinical clues about being in direct contact with foliage and the fact that only the uncovered parts of the body were affected. The difficult part is remembering what type of hypersensitivity reaction poison ivy or poison provokes, which is actually a type 4 (cell-mediated) reaction. Be sure to remember these types of questions as they may also be on your Pediatrics shelf as well.

      A. Hypersensitivity, type 1 → Incorrect. This is an IgE-mediated reaction that is often manifested by allergic responses.

      B. Hypersensitivity, type 2 → Incorrect. This is an antibody-mediated reaction that is often times seen with blood type (ABO) incompatibility.

      C. Hypersensitivity, type 3 → Incorrect. This is an immune complex-mediated reaction (IgG and IgM, in particular) to blood containing pre-formed antibodies or with particular drugs.

      E. Jarisch-Herxheimer reaction → Incorrect. There was no indication that a patient has taken an antibiotic for his troubles.

2. WWGJD: A 29-year-old female with a history of HIV for 5 years comes to the physician for a follow-up appointment. She endorses being compliant with the medication and having no trouble controlling her symptoms. She is currently taking the HAART regimen and a proton pump inhibitor for GERD. CD4 counts that were last checked indicate that she was near normal. She does however, **endorse being around people who cough all the time recently, from her significant other to her parents who live nearby. What is the next most appropriate step?**

Answer: C, PPD skin test.

Explanation: It is recommended that all HIV patients at some point get tested for tuberculosis, since those two diseases are so intertwined. Thus, the first step in prophylaxis is to try to rule out TB early. PPD is the fastest and most cost-effective way to do so.

A. Reassurance → Incorrect. While reassurance may feel good for the patient, she still needs a PPD to rule out TB.

B. Prescribe anxiolytic → Incorrect. It is never appropriate to prescribe an anxiolytic without the proper indication. In this case, there was no indication the patient had pathologic worry (e.g., sleep disturbances, disturbance of daily activities).

D. Spirometry → Incorrect. No need for spirometry here, although may have use in patients with chronic disorders of the respiratory system, such as cystic fibrosis.

E. Chest X-ray → Incorrect. Although may be tempting to rule out pneumonia, it is important to recognize that the patient herself is NOT coughing; she only complains about all the people around her who do. Thus, at this moment, she does not have respiratory pathology and would best be suited by administering the PPD.

Diseases of the Blood and Blood-Forming Organs

Leo Wang, Sila Bal, Kaitlyn Barkley, Hao-Hua Wu, and Katherine Margo

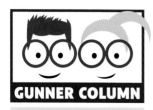

GUNNER COLUMN

Introduction

This chapter covers the hematology/oncology that you will face on the family medicine shelf. The chapter is low yield and only makes up 1%–5% of the family medicine shelf. Whereas almost any content from the medicine shelf is fair game for the family medicine shelf, the family medicine shelf will focus specifically on prophylaxis, diagnosis, and outpatient treatment and management.

This chapter is divided into several subsections that highlight the various pathologies that can occur in the blood, ranging from infections to clotting problems to cancer. As a rule, complete blood counts (CBCs) and peripheral blood smears can play major diagnostic roles in the workup of many of these diseases. The analysis of these CBCs and peripheral smears are less emphasized, but you should still recognize that these need to be ordered. For specific diseases such as coagulopathies, understanding principles behind PT, aPTT (discussed later) will be helpful but not necessary

Infections of the Blood and Lymph

This chapter covers various types of infections of the blood and lymphatic system. The concepts applied herein are relatively general. On the family medicine shelf, focus specifically on **prophylaxis** and **diagnosis**. There are a few key treatment modalities, which we have highlighted. The **single most important infection of the blood** is HIV/AIDS. You must know this disease in great detail for the family medicine shelf.

Malaria

Buzz Words: Cyclical/irregular fevers (e.g., fever every 48–72 hours) + anemia + jaundice + splenomegaly + endemic area (Africa)

Clinical Presentation: Malaria is a mosquito-borne disease caused by a parasite of the *Plasmodium* species. The most common cause of death is by *Plasmodium falciparum*, as vivax, ovale, and malariae cause mild disease. Malaria replicates in RBCs, leading to a hemolytic anemia. A classical finding in malaria is paroxysm, where cold/shivers alternate with fever/sweating that repeats every 2 days. Initial infection with malaria is usually severe; individuals can get immunity and get milder infections as they age. Family medicine physicians in the United States will not see many patients presenting with malaria, but family medicine physicians abroad may see this frequently.

Prophylactic (PPx): (1) Mosquito control; (2) doxycycline, mefloquine, atovaquone/proguanil—plasmodium-resistant species; (3) chloroquine/hydroxychloroquine—plasmodium sensitive species; (4) dapsone/primaquine/quinine

Mechanism of Disease (MoD): Infected *Anopheles* female mosquito transmits malaria sporozoites to humans through the bloodstream, which travel to the liver for a 2-week incubation period. Symptoms begin after 2–4 weeks; if infected with *Plasmodium vivax* and *Plasmodium ovale*, patients may get symptoms months after exposure due to activation of hypnozoites in the liver.

Diagnostic Steps (Dx):
1. Recent travel history
2. CBC
3. Giemsa-stained blood smear
4. Antigen rapid detection tests

Treatment/Management (Tx/Mgmt):
1. Chloroquine
2. In resistant areas use artemisinin combination therapy (ACT) or atovaquone-proguanil
3. Quinine and mefloquine

Human Immunodeficiency Virus Infection and Acquired Immunodeficiency Syndrome

Buzz Words: Sexually active male or female + intravenous (IV) drug user + enlarged inguinal lymph nodes (or generalized lymphadenopathy) + fever/recent sickness + sore throat + unspecified rashes → HIV (acute phase)

Toxoplasma infection + *Cryptosporidium* infection, *Mycobacterium avium* infection, fungal infections (*Candida, Cryptococcus, Pneumocysitis, Histoplasma, Coccidioides*) + cytomegalovirus (CMV) + Kaposi's sarcoma + lymphomas + encephalopathy + wasting syndrome → Manifestations of acquired immune deficiency syndrome (AIDS when CD4 <200 and considered late phase of infection)

Clinical Presentation: HIV is a double-stranded RNA virus that infects immune cells (e.g., CD4) by embedding themselves into DNA through reverse transcription. On the family medicine shelf, patients can either present in the acute phase of illness (e.g., sore throat, generalized lymphadenopathy, fever) or late stage of illness aka with acquired immunodeficiency syndrome.

For the Family Medicine exam, make sure to know the screening guidelines for HIV:

1. All men and women 15–65 years old should be screened
2. All men and women who seek evaluation or treatment for sexually transmitted infections (STIs) should be screened
3. All pregnant women should be screened at the first prenatal visit
4. Men who have sex with men (MSM) should be screened annually

PPx: To understand prophylactic measures, know the common modes of HIV transmission: (1) sexual intercourse through genital, rectal, or oral fluids; (2) use of contaminated instruments or needles (e.g., IV drug users sharing needles); (3) maternal to fetus through breastfeeding or childbirth; and (4) blood transfusion. Thus, to prevent HIV transmission: (1) condom use, (2) avoidance of dirty needles, (3) treatment of pregnant patient to reduce HIV viral load and chance of vertical transmission, (4) screening of blood donors for HIV, (5) HIV antibody testing for sexually active patients, (6) stay updated with vaccinations (flu, hepatitis B virus [HBV], pneumococcal, human papillomavirus [HPV], zoster).

MoD: HIV is a lentivirus capable of long-term latent infection and spread through semen and blood → HIV Env (envelope glycoprotein) binds to CD4 and chemokine coreceptors (CXCR4, CCR5) → HIV RNA w/ reverse transcriptase release into cell → HIV integration into genome and replication within cell → lysis of infected cell to release of HIV and propagate infection.

HIV infection leads to immunodeficiency by (1) loss of CD4 cells from direct cytotoxic effect; (2) infection of macrophages, dendritic cells, and follicular dendritic cells; (3) decreased immune response caused by depletion of CD4 T cells.

Dx:
1. HIV antibody testing
2. Nucleic acid amplification assays for HIV RNA level
3. ELISA ± Western blot to confirm diagnosis
- To monitor HIV, order:
  1. CD4 count (e.g., CBC with diff)
  2. Plasma HIV RNA level

   3. PPD or quantiferon gold to r/o concomitant tuber-
      culosis (TB)

Tx/Mgmt:
1. Combination treatment with antiretroviral therapy, for
   example, highly active antiretroviral therapy (HAART)
2. If AIDS (CD4 <200 μL), TMP/SMX or dapsone to PPx
   against *P. jiroveci*
3. If AIDS (CD4 <50), azithromycin/clarithromycin to PPx
   against *Mycobacterium avium-intracellulare* (MAC)
4. If HIV + suspicion of TB, start patient on isoniazid and
   pyridoxine (vitamin B6 to counter isoniazid side effects)
5. If worry for fungal infections, fluconazole

Cat Scratch Disease (Bartonella henselae)

Buzz Words: Tender + swollen lymph nodes occurring near
   site of bite or scratch from cat + generalized malaise

Clinical Presentation: This is an infection by a Gram-negative
   bacillus that you get from scratches from a flea-infested
   cat. Commonly found in children. In very rare cases,
   cat scratch disease can cause meningitis, encephalitis, endocarditis, and other very mortal complications. Immunocompromised patients may get bacillary
   angiomatosis or bacillary peliosis.

PPx: (1) Take flea control measures after handling cat/feces

MoD: Systemic symptoms caused by widespread dissemination of *B. henselae* following inoculation (most
   commonly cat scratch). Can also lead to lymphadenitis.

Dx:
1. Blood cultures
2. Polymerase chain reaction (PCR)
3. Clinical
4. Warthin-Starry stain (microbial cultures)

Tx/Mgmt:
1. Emergency room referral based on exam findings
2. Azithromycin, doxycycline, or ciprofloxacin

Anemias

Anemia should be approached systematically as microcytic (MCV <80), macrocytic (MCV >100), and normocytic
anemias, corresponding to small, large, and normal-
sized RBCs, respectively. For the family medicine shelf,
again focus on being able to recognize anemia from
the buzz words and clinical presentation and the basic
diagnostic methodologies to distinguish between them
(Fig. 4.1).

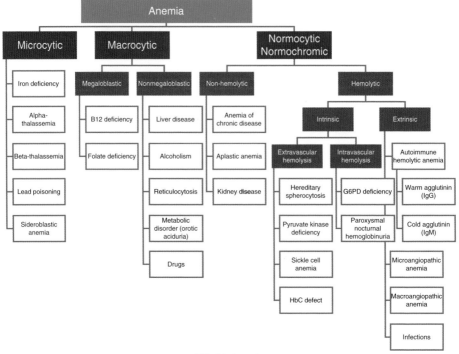

FIG. 4.1 Anemia.

Iron Deficiency Anemia

Buzz Words: Fatigue + dizziness + pallor + microcytic anemia + low ferritin + low reticulocyte count + increased total iron-binding capacity (TIBC) → iron deficiency anemia

Pica + koilonychias (concave nails) + cheilosis + glossitis → severe iron deficiency anemia

Clinical Presentation: Iron deficiency is the most common cause of anemia and more likely to be found in females (especially those who are pregnant), infants, and the elderly. Suspect in female patients who present with a chief complaint of fatigue. In elderly patients, suspect occult blood loss until otherwise proven (e.g., melena or peptic ulcer disease).

PPx: (1) No screening recommended by the USPSTF, (2) counseling about foods that contain iron

MoD: Variable but can be most commonly due to insufficient intake and blood loss. Can also be due to increased iron requirement (e.g., infants, pregnancy) or decreased iron absorption (e.g., celiac disease, gastrectomy).

Dx:

1. CBC
2. Peripheral blood smear

99 AR

The most current USPSTF guidelines that pregnant women and children between the age of 6 and 12 months do NOT have to be screened. This is a departure from their old guidelines that did recommend for screening. Keep this in mind as you may read texts that are out of date.

3. Iron studies (iron, TIBC, ferritin, transferrin, reticulocyte count, red cell distribution width)

Tx/Mgmt:
1. Oral supplemental iron
2. Parenteral iron

Anemia of Chronic Disease (Inflammation)

Buzz Words: Microcytic or normocytic anemia + elevated ferritin + decreased Fe/TIBC + malignancy + autoimmune conditions

Clinical Presentation: Microcytic or normocytic anemia with elevated ferritin (storage form of iron) but decreased serum iron levels. TIBC decreased. Can be seen in the setting of malignancy and autoimmune conditions. Patients will present with fatigue, weakness, pallor in setting of autoimmune disorders, endocarditis, malignancy.

PPx: N/A

MoD: Chronic disease state → elevated acute phase reactants (hepcidin) → hepcidin pushes iron into storage form in order to prevent bacterial access to iron → decreased free iron causes decreased hemoglobin production → microcytic anemia.

Dx:
1. CBC
2. Peripheral blood smear
3. Iron studies
4. Acute phase reactants (elevated hepcidin)

Tx/Mgmt:
1. Treat underlying cause, otherwise, no treatment for asymptomatic anemia
2. EPO if symptomatic
3. Transfusion if severely decreased hemoglobin

Thalassemias

Buzz Words: Target cells + Mediterranean descent → beta thalassemia

HbA2 + HbBarts/HbH + Southeast Asian → alpha thalassemia

Clinical Presentation: Thalassemias are a microcytic anemia of varying severity. In severe cases, patients may exhibit signs of extramedullary hematopoiesis with a crew-cut appearance of skull on X-ray, chipmunk facies due to facial bone involvement, and hepatosplenomegaly. Thalassemias generally present a few months after birth as HbF is protective.

PPx: (1) Screening for beta-thalassemia included in the uniform screening panel; otherwise no specific screening recommendations

MoD: The major hemoglobin found in adults is hemoglobin A, composed of 2 alpha and 2 beta chains. Thalassemia is an inherited mutation in the alpha or beta globin chain of hemoglobin resulting in decreased hemoglobin synthesis. Both forms lead to increased hemolysis and extramedullary hematopoiesis with resultant enlarged bones.

- Alpha thalassemia is more commonly seen in Southeast Asian populations with four variations:
  - One–two gene deletions result in normal or mild anemia.
  - Three gene deletions result in Barts (HgH) disease: severe anemia with a chain that binds strongly to oxygen similar to fetal Hb.
  - Four gene deletions are unsustainable with life, resulting in hydrops fetalis.
- Beta thalassemia is more commonly seen in Mediterranean populations:
  - Heterozygotes will have beta thalassemia minor and present with mild microcytic anemia.
  - Homozygotes will have Cooleys anemia with hepatosplenomegaly, bone marrow hyperplasia with thalassemia face. These patients may require lifelong transfusions resulting in secondary hemochromatosis (iron overload).

Dx:
1. CBC
2. Hemoglobin electrophoresis with **HbA2 or HbF and little/no HbA**
3. Peripheral smear shows microcytic, hypochromic RBCs with target cells

Tx/Mgmt:
1. Observation if asymptomatic
2. Iron supplementation for hemolysis
3. Blood transfusions

TABLE 4.1 Lab Values for Iron Deficiency Anemia, Anemia of Chronic Disease, and Thalassemia

	Iron	Ferritin	TIBC
Iron deficiency anemia	Low	Low	High
Anemia of chronic disease	Low	High	Low
Thalassemia	Normal or high	Normal or high	Normal

TIBC, Total iron-binding capacity.

Vitamin B12 (Cobalamin) Deficiency

Buzz Words: Macrocytic anemia + gastrointestinal (GI) symptoms + weakness + spasticity + absent reflexes + diminished vibration and position sensation + subacute degeneration of spinal cord + memory loss + depression

Clinical Presentation: Vitamin B12 deficiency is also known as subacute combined degeneration of the spinal cord that presents with posterior and lateral column signs. It can also cause macrocyctic anemia.

PPx: (1) B12 supplementation, diet including animal products

MoD: (1) Decreased B12 → Impaired DNA synthesis and regulation, fatty acid and amino acid metabolism

Dx:
1. Labs → Vitamin B12 levels with elevated methylmalonic acid levels
2. Anti-intrinsic factor antibodies to r/o pernicious anemia

Tx/Mgmt:
1. Vitamin B12 supplementation

> **QUICK TIPS**
>
> B12 versus folate deficiency: There are no neurologic symptoms in folate deficiency.

Sickle Cell Disease

Sickle cell is a commonly tested hematologic disease that appears on every standardized exam available, including the family medicine shelf.

Buzz Words: Painful fingers and toes in young African-American children + fatigue, pallor + shortness of breath (acute chest) + familial pattern + splenic atrophy

Clinical Presentation: Sickle cell is an autosomal recessive trait that causes the formation of hemoglobin S. Hemoglobin S is prone to "sickling" under low oxygen states, which leads to a plethora of complications that arise from hemolysis and sickling in inappropriate places. **Vaso-occlusion can** occur when sickled RBCs obstruct capillary beds and lead to ischemia, infarction, and necrosis of organs. One of the most commonly infarcted organs is the spleen, which will lead to splenic atrophy. Many sickle cell patients are therefore functional asplenics. Lack of spleen function renders these patients susceptible to encapsulated organisms, most commonly *Streptococcus pneumoniae* and *Haemophilus influenzae*. In some cases, splenic sequestration can occur, where sickled cells get sequestered in the spleen, leading to huge falls in hemoglobin and eventual circulatory failure. Acute chest syndrome is a common finding in patients with sickle-cell disease (SCD), where sickled RBCs occlude the capillaries in the lungs leading to respiratory compromise and hypoxemia. Dactylitis is an early finding in patients with sickle cell, which is characterized by painful fingers and toes due to sickled RBC

gg AR

Uniform screening panel recommended by US Department of Health and Human Services

occlusion of their vasculature. Sickle cell patients can also have aplastic crises, where an infection by parvovirus B19 (or other agents) leads to rapid degradation of RBCs, leading to abrupt declines in RBC count that can be life threatening. Other complications of sickle cell include priapism, cholelithiasis (bilirubin breakdown → gallstones), stroke, renal papillary necrosis, ulcers, osteomyelitis pulmonary hypertension → right heart failure, and opioid tolerance and addiction. Frequently ask yourself why each of these complications happen as a means to better learn them. The precipitant behind everything anyone can get from sickle cell is **vaso-occlusion and hemolysis.**

PPx: 1. Screening for sickle cell included in uniform screening panel; 2. daily penicillin prophylaxis as child for *S. pneumoniae;* 3. vaccination for *S. pneumoniae, H. influenzae,* meningococcus; 4. anti-malarial chemoprophylaxis in areas endemic; 5. counseling for parents with sickle trait/disease

MoD: Glutamic acid (hydrophilic) to valine (hydrophobic) substitution of the beta-globin gene leads to sickling (hydrophobic amino acids like to aggregate) inherited in autosomal recessive fashion. Oxygen tension normally leads to high elasticity, allowing RBCs to pass through capillary beds. In sickled states, oxygen tension is unable to enhance RBC elasticity due to the aggregated, sickled beta-globin. This leads to hemolysis and vaso-occlusive crises.

Dx:
1. CBC; low Hb, high reticulocyte count
2. Sodium metabisulfite-induced RBC sickling
3. Hb electrophoresis
4. UA, UCx, CXR, blood cultures for infection workup

Tx/Mgmt:
1. Folic acid
2. Patient-controlled analgesia for vaso-occlusion
3. Oxygen supplementation, transfusion for acute chest crisis
4. **Hydroxyurea** → elevated HbF production (fetal hemoglobin has higher affinity for O_2)
5. Blood transfusions
6. Bone marrow transplant (curative)

Coagulation Disorders

You will likely have at least one question on coagulation disorders on the family medicine shelf. The most commonly tested topics are hemophilia, von Willebrand disease and antiphospholipid syndrome.

As an organizing principle, most coagulopathies are diagnosed from CBC, PT, aPTT, and bleeding times. Treatments should be commensurate with the underlying pathologies, which should be anticoagulants in hypercoagulable states, and pro-coagulants in hypocoagulable states. This should be intuitive.

Hemophilia A

Buzz Words: Knee joint bleeding at early age + intracranial bleeding + hematuria + familial pattern

Clinical Presentation: X-linked recessive disorder from missing factor VIII. The most common sign is joint bleeding, also known as hemarthrosis, which can lead to joint destruction. However, bleeding can occur in other areas, and the most common cause of death in these patients is intracranial bleeding.

PPx: Prevent trauma

MoD: Deficiency in factor VIII leads to defect in intrinsic pathway → hypocoagulability.

Dx:
1. CBC
2. PT/aPTT
   - Prolonged PTT
3. Low factor VIII levels and normal von Willebrand disease (vWF)

Tx/Mgmt:
1. Analgesia and immobilization for acute hermarthrosis
2. FVIII replacement
3. DDAVP → leads to endothelial secretion of vWF, which is a carrier for FVIII and protects it

Hemophilia B

Buzz Words: Knee joint bleeding at early age + intracranial bleeding + hematuria + familial pattern

Clinical Presentation: X-linked recessive disorder; rarer than hemophilia A but presents identically. Caused by deficiency in factor IX.

PPx: Prevent trauma

MoD: Deficiency in factor IX leads to defect in intrinsic pathway → hypocoagulability

Dx:
1. CBC
2. PT/aPTT
   - Prolonged PTT
3. Low VIII levels

Tx/Mgmt:
1. Analgesia and immobilization for acute hemarthrosis
2. FVIII replacement

von Willebrand Disease

Buzz Words: Recurrent nosebleeds + cutaneous bleeding + gingival bleeding + bleeding after dental procedures + menorrhagia + GI bleeding + elevated bleeding time

Clinical Presentation: vWF disease is a common, autosomal dominant disease leading to deficiency in vWF. vWF plays two roles: it binds to platelets to allow them to adhere to vessel walls, and is a carrier for factor VIII that prevents it from degradation. Thus, vWF plays two pro-coagulant roles that when missing leads to a hypocoagulable state. There are three kinds in order from most to least common:
Type 1—decreased levels
Type 2—dysfunctional, but normal levels
Type 3—missing vWF (severe)

PPx: Avoid aspirin/nonsteroidal anti-inflammatory drugs (NSAIDs) → overbleeding

MoD: vWF is secreted from megakaryocytes and endothelial cells that protects FVIII in the blood from degradation and is also part of aggregating platelets by allowing them to adhere to endothelial cells after injury. In vWF, vWF is missing or defective, leading to an inability for platelets to aggregate and for FVIII to partake in the coagulation cascade. This leads to problems primarily with mucosal bleeding, where the most common sign is recurrent nosebleeds (epistaxis).

Dx:
1. CBC
2. PT/aPTT
3. Elevated bleeding time
4. Decreased vWF and factor VIII activity
5. Ristocetin platelet aggregation
   a. Platelets will not aggregate

Tx/Mgmt:
1. DDAVP—causes endothelial cells to secrete vWF
2. Factor VIII concentrates

Antiphospholipid Syndrome (Lupus Anticoagulant, Anticardiolipin)

Buzz Words: Repeat arterial and venous thromboses + stroke/TIA + lupus + intrauterine death or intrauterine growth restriction + placental infarctions

Clinical Presentation: Antiphospholipid antibodies lead to recurrent venous/arterial thromboses, presenting with complications like recurrent deep vein thrombosis (DVT)/PE, stroke, and other conditions. A common presenting finding is a pregnancy complication, such as intrauterine death. APLS is categorized into primary versus secondary. Primary APLS is idiopathic in nature. Secondary APLS is caused by conditions like lupus.

PPx: N/A

MoD: Phospholipids are part of all cell membranes. Antiphospholipid antibodies are antibodies made against these components of all cell membranes. Sometimes these phospholipids take on specific names, like cardiolipin. Anticardiolipin antibodies are antibodies toward a specific phospholipid in the mitochondrial (and hence they are also anti-mitochondrial) and are elevated in diseases including SLE and syphilis. These bind to ApoH, activating it leading to inhibition of protein C. Protein C is then unable to exert its anticoagulant effect on the clotting cascade. Lupus anticoagulant is an antiphospholipid that binds to prothrombin, activating it to form thrombin leading to a pro-coagulant state. They also target beta-2microgbulin, which also leads to thrombosis. The lupus anticoagulant is a PRO-coagulant in vivo despite its name. It receives its name for its function in vitro, where it increases PTT.

QUICK TIPS
Another confusing part of the lupus anticoagulant is that most people with it actually don't have lupus.

Dx:
1. CBC
2. PT/aPTT
3. Mixing test
   a. Lupus anticoagulant will inhibit clotting in normal plasma
4. Serological testing (ELISA)

Tx/Mgmt:
1. Observation
2. Lifelong anticoagulation

GUNNER PRACTICE

1. A woman presents to her physician prior to traveling to many locations in Africa for a vacation. She is not pregnant and not sexually active. She has no past medical history. Which of the following is appropriate prophylaxis?
   A. No chemoprophylaxis
   B. Chloroquine
   C. Mefloquine
   D. Doxycycline
   E. Azithromycin

2. An 18-year-old female presents to her doctor with a sore throat for 1 week. Her throat is especially sore with swallowing. She has been having fevers and fatigue as well. She has not been attending practice for field hockey secondary to not feeling well. She did get her flu shot at school 3 weeks prior to symptom onset. On exam her vital signs are normal. Her throat shows tonsillar erythema and edema with bilateral exudates. Her exam is otherwise normal. Rapid strep test is negative. What is the next best step?

A. Reassurance
B. Mono spot test
C. Strep culture
D. Initiate antibiotics for strep pharyngitis
E. Tonsillectomy

3. A 16-year-old female presents to her family doctor for fatigue and weight loss. She has lost 12 pounds over 3 months and her body mass index (BMI) is now 18.5. On exam she has tachycardia with pallor. She has no lymphadenopathy. The results of her CBC is shown below. Which of the following is most likely?

Hemoglobin	6.7	(g/dL)
WBC	63.8	($\times 10^9$/L)
Neutrophils	19.2	($\times 10^9$/L)
Platelets	53	($\times 10^9$/L)

A. ALL
B. APL
C. AML
D. CML
E. CLL

Notes

ANSWERS: What Would Gunner Jess/Jim Do?

1. **WWGJD?** A woman presents to her physician prior to traveling to many locations in **Africa for a vacation.** She is not pregnant and not sexually active. She has no past medical history. Which of the following is appropriate **prophylaxis?**

   Answer: C

   The question is very vague about where the woman is traveling. The questions on the shelf may be more specific. The CDC and WHO recommendations about chemoprophylaxis for malaria are constantly being updated, which makes answering these questions challenging. It is safe to assume that in this question, the woman is traveling to areas where malaria is chloroquine resistant. In that case, mefloquine is the ideal agent. Doxycycline can be used for prophylaxis but causes a terrible rash when the patient is exposed to sun, which makes it less ideal than mefloquine. Azithromycin is not used for malaria prophylaxis.

2. **WWGJD?** An 18-year-old female presents to her doctor with **a sore throat for 1 week.** Her throat is especially sore with swallowing. She has been having **fevers and fatigue** as well. She has not been attending practice for **field hockey** secondary to not feeling well. She did get her flu shot at school 3 weeks prior to symptom onset. On exam her vital signs are normal. Her throat shows **tonsillar erythema and edema with bilateral exudates.** Her exam is otherwise normal. **Rapid strep test is negative.** What is the next best step?

   Answer: B

   This patient has mononucleosis. Since she plays a contact sport, it is important to diagnose the disease. If the mono spot test is positive, she should avoid playing field hockey so as to not risk damage to her spleen, which is likely enlarged even though the question stem did not mention it. Answer A may be appropriate in a child who does not play contact sports. Answers C and D would be appropriate if the strep test was positive. Answer E is probably never the correct answer. It is very invasive and not an appropriate next step unless the tonsils are occluding the airway. Even then, the next step would be to intubate, not to remove the tonsils.

3. **WWGJD?** A 16-year-old female presents to her family doctor for fatigue and weight loss. She has lost 12

pounds over 3 months and her BMI is now 18.5. On exam she has tachycardia with pallor. She has no lymphadenopathy. The results of her CBC is shown below. Which of the following is most likely?

Hemoglobin	6.7	(g/dL)
WBC	63.8	($\times 10^9$/L)
Neutrophils	10.2	($\times 10^9$/L)
Platelets	53	($\times 10^9$/L)

Answer A

ALL stands for acute lymphoblastic leukemia. It is a common cancer in childhood and often presents as in the question stem. When given lab values on the shelf exam, you can usually ignore the question stem and answer the question from the lab values. The only information that matters in the question stem here is the age of the patient. The CBC shows a massive leukocytosis which suggests leukemia. The leukocytes are not neutrophil predominant, which is suggestive of a lymphoid as opposed to myeloid leukemia. So, answers B, C, and D can be ruled out. Note that APL is a specific type of AML. CLL is chronic lymphocytic leukemia and is very rare in patients under 60 years of age. This makes answer A the best answer.

Mental Disorders

*Isabella Bellon, Leo Wang, Hao-Hua Wu, and
Katherine Margo*

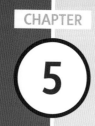

Introduction

Mental disorders are extremely common in both the primary care setting as well as your family medicine shelf exam. In family medicine, common things being common, the scope of mental disorders that are tested on the shelf exam can be largely separated as follows: mood disorders and anxiety disorders. Other salient topics in primary care include substance use disorders and suicide screening, both of which will also be discussed here.

This chapter will be divided into four main sections. First, the mood disorders will be discussed. These disorders are characterized by abnormal depression or elevation of a person's mood and include major depression disorder, dysthymia, adjustment disorder, bipolar disorder, and cyclothymic disorder.

Second, the anxiety disorders will be discussed. These disorders are characterized by excessive worry and fear and include generalized anxiety disorder, panic disorder (PD), obsessive-compulsive disorder (OCD), posttraumatic stress disorder (PTSD), and phobias (specific and social).

The third and fourth sections will be brief and provide an overview of the substance use disorder with an emphasis on outlining the difference between substance abuse and substance dependence. The chapter will conclude with a brief, yet important, note on suicide risk factors and screening.

Mental Disorders

Mood Disorders

The way to approach mood starts by teasing out whether one's symptoms are depressive, manic, or hypomanic episode. Once you've determined this distinction, you should then look at the time list of symptoms to help you land at a Diagnostic Steps (Dx). Before we address each of the mood disorders and how they are associated with the presence of different episodes, you should focus on learning how to diagnose each type of episode. Follow the structure below to be able to make such distinction.

Major Depressive Episode

- Use the mnemonic SIGECAPS. A patient will meet criteria for a depressive episode if he or she exhibits four of the listed symptoms in addition to having depressed mood or anhedonia (aka 5/9 of the SIGECAPS). Symptoms must be present for 2 weeks and cause social or occupational impairment.
- Symptoms cannot be due to substance use or other medical condition.
- SIGECAPS:
  - **S**leep (insomnia or hypersomnia)
  - Loss of **I**nterest
  - **G**uilt
  - Low **E**nergy
  - Impaired **C**oncentration
  - Change in **A**ppetite
  - **P**sychomotor retardation or agitation
  - **S**uicidal thoughts

Manic Episode

- Use the mnemonic DIG FAST. Patient will meet criteria if he or she has had three or more of the following symptoms for at least 1 week and must cause social and occupational impairment. Once again, symptoms should not be associated with substance use.
- DIG FAST:
  - **D**istractibility and easy frustration
  - **I**rresponsibility and uninhibited behavior
  - **G**randiosity
  - **F**light of ideas
  - **A**ctivity increased with weight loss and increased libido
  - **S**leep need decreased
  - **T**alkativeness/pressured speech

Hypomanic Episode

- The patient will have elevated, expansive, or irritable mood with at least three of the DIG FAST symptoms lasting more than 4 days and WITHOUT marked social or occupational impairment.

  Now that you know how distinguish episodes, use the following guide to arrive at the correct Dx:

A. Major Depressive Disorder

Buzz Words: >1 depressive episode (depressed mood or loss of interest or pleasure + 4 SIGECAPS + >2 weeks) + (female > male or elderly)

QUICK TIPS

It can be difficult to distinguish between mania and hypomania. Episodes that are associated with psychosis, marked vocational/social impairment, or require hospitalization are manic. Hypomania can be short-lived and does not necessarily interfere with daily life.

Clinical Presentation: Age: Average onset mid-20s, increased incidence among elderly

Gender: 2× more prevalent in females (female:male equal among elderly)

Site of care: Outpatient

Chief Complaint: Patients may report sadness, negative thinking, hopelessness, worthlessness as well as irritability or mood swings. Somatic complaints of decreased energy and difficulty concentrating are common. Elderly may present with confusion and general decline in functioning.

PMH/PSuH/PFH/PSoH: Family history of depression/anxiety (2–3× more likely to develop depression). Comorbidity with anxiety and substance use disorders is common.

Prophylactic (PPx): None

Mechanism of Disease (MoD): Etiology is thought to be multifactorial involving genetic, biology, environment, and psychosocial factors. Leading theory states that depression is caused by neurotransmitter deficiencies in the brain. This theory is supported by the fact that antidepressants that increase the availability of serotonin, norepinephrine, and dopamine alleviate depressive symptoms.

Dx:

1. Rule out medical disorders that mimic depressive symptom (hypothyroidism, anemia, infection/human immunodeficiency virus, cancer).
2. Rule out other mood disorders (dysthymia, bereavement, and bipolar disorder).
3. Recent medication changes (beta-blockers, steroids, sedatives).
4. Inquire about substance use, abuse or dependence (alcohol, narcotics, cocaine).
5. Address suicidal ideations.

PHQ2 questions: Over the past 2 weeks, have you been bothered by the following?

1. Little interest or pleasure in doing things
2. Feeling down, depressed, or hopeless

https://se.pinterest.com/pin/4011087142906967/

Treatment/Management (Tx/Mgmt):

1. Psychotherapy and pharmacotherapy together are better than either regimen alone.
2. No class of medication has been proven to be more effective.

QUICK TIPS

PHQ2 and PHQ9 are tools used to assess depression. If a patient answers "yes" to either question on the PHQ2 assessment tool, administer the PHQ9.

FOR THE WARDS

SSRIs may be used during pregnancy as they have not been shown to increase risk of major malformation, miscarriage, stillbirth, or prematurity. Hold off during 1st trimester.

3. Antidepressant effect may take 4–6 weeks after onset of therapy.
4. Treated for 6–12 months and then reassess. Long-term (2 years or lifelong) treatment is recommended for patient with a history of three or more major depressive episodes.
5. Treatment failure most commonly due to underdosing, poor adherence, and not allowing enough time for full effect of medications.

Pharmacotherapy

Class	Medication	Side Effects	Comments
SSRI—Selective serotonin reuptake inhibitor	Fluoxetine Paroxetine Sertraline Citalopram Escitalopram Flucoxamine	Headache, GI disturbance, sexual dysfunction, rebound anxiety	Most common agents used
SNRI— Serotonin and Norepinephrine reuptake inhibitor	Venlafaxine Desvenlafaxine Duloxetine	Nausea, dizziness, sweating, sexual dysfunction, tiredness	
TCA—Tricyclic antidepressant	Amitriptyline Nortriptyline Desipramine Clomipramine Doxepin Imipramine	Sedation, weight gain, orthostatic hypotension, anticholinergic effects, increase QTc	Potential for lethal overdose
Atypicals	Bupropion Mirtazapine Trazodone	→ Contraindicated in anorexia → Sedation → Very sedating and priapism	Buproprion is a norepinephrine and dopamine reuptake inhibitor
MAOI— Monoamine oxidase inhibitor	Phenelzine Tranylcypromine	Orthostatic hypotension Hypertensive crisis when combined with tyramine-rich foods (wine, beer, aged cheeses) Risk of serotonin syndrome if taken with SSRI	Useful in refractory depression

B. Dysthymic Disorder

Buzz Words: Low mood + >2 (changes in appetite, changes in sleep, low self-esteem, poor concentration, low energy, feelings of hopelessness) + 2 years

Clinical Presentation: Age: All ages, but most prevalent amongst the elderly

Gender: Females > males

Site of care: Outpatient

Chief Complaint: Low energy, negative outlook on life. Diurnal variation may also be present (patient will report more symptoms in the morning, for example).

PMH/PSuH/PFH/PSoH: Family history of mood disorders increases risk. Patient may report spending most of his or her energy on work and leaving little room for socializing and family life.

PPx: None

MoD: Multifactorial, genetic, biology, social stressors, medical problems, poor coping strategies all seem to play a role. Neurotransmitter dysfunctions (serotonin and norepinephrine) have been implicated given response to antidepressants.

Dx:

1. Similar to major depressive disorder (MDD), rule thyroid pathology.
2. Evaluate for substance use as well as other mood disorders.

Tx/Mgmt: Psychotherapy and medical management with SSRI, SNRIs, and TCA (see above)

C. Adjustment Disorder

Buzz Words: Identifiable stressor + emotional/behavioral symptoms that are out of proportion to intensity of stressor ± functional impairment within 3–6 months from stressor onset.

Clinical Presentation: Age: Most common in adolescence, but can happen at any age

Gender: 2:1, female:male

Site of care: Outpatient

Chief Complaint: May be vague and include poor sleep, poor concentration, low mood, and anxiety in the setting of a recent stressor.

PMH/PSuH/PFH/PSoH: Previous Dx with mood or personality disorders, substance abuse, or organic mental disorders increase risk of developing adjustment disorder.

PPx: None

MoD: Unclear etiology. Multifactorial, involving a combination of genetic, environmental, developmental, preexisting personality traits, past personal history, and coping skills. Adjustment disorder is considered an **anxiety disorder** by mechanism and thus is not treated like other mood disorders.

Dx:

1. Complete a mental status examination.
2. Evaluate for suicide and homicide.
3. Hallucinations or delusions denote psychotic process.

Tx/Mgmt: Psychotherapy (supportive or group) preferred given adjustment disorder tendency to be a short-term disorder. May provide pharmacotherapy for associated symptoms such as insomnia, anxiety, or depression.

D. Bipolar Disorder, Type I

Buzz Words (Bipolar I): One manic episode

Clinical Presentation: Age: ~20 years old (90% of patients are diagnosed before age 30)

Gender: Female = male

Site of care: Outpatient

Chief Complaint: Most patients present with complaints associated with depressive episodes (low mood, low energy, changes in sleep, etc.). Patients rarely present during a manic episode given mania is often not perceived as an illness.

PMH/PSuH/PFH/PSoH: Highly heritable and related to multiple genes.

MoD: Pathophysiology has yet to be determined, and etiology seems to be multifactorial including genetic, biochemical, psychosocial, and environmental factors.

Dx:

1. Rule out substance use.
2. Clinical Dx; however, keep in mind that medical problems including hyper- and hypothyroidism, Cushing disease, neurosyphilis, and Lyme disease should be part of the differential Dx.

Tx/Mgmt:

1. Lithium and valproate are first-line (but avoid lithium in patients with poor renal function).
2. Use valproate or carbamazepine in a patient with mixed or rapid cycling episodes.

QUICK TIPS

Note that bereavement is the term used to describe symptoms such as (crying spells, problem sleeping, trouble concentrating) associated with the death of a loved one. If symptoms last for longer than 2 months and include psychosis or suicidal ideation, then a Dx of MDD is made.

QUICK TIPS

First-degree relatives at 7–10× more likely to develop mania, and 2× more likely to develop depression.

QUICK TIPS

Bipolar I has the highest genetic link of all major psychiatric disorders.

3. Atypical antipsychotics (olanzapine, quetiapine, ziprasidone) are effective as both monotherapy and adjunct therapy for acute mania.
   • Avoid antidepressants as they may induce a manic episode.

E. Bipolar Disorder, Type II

Buzz Words (Bipolar II): Milder symptoms than type I, at least one major depressive episode + hypomanic episode

Clinical Presentation: Age: Onset before 30 years of age

Gender: Women > men

Site of care: Outpatient

Chief Complaint: As noted above, complaints are often associated with depressive symptoms.

PMH/PSuH/PFH/PSoH: Same as bipolar I (see above)

PPx: None

MoD: Same as bipolar type I (see above)

Dx:

1. Rule out substance use.
2. Clinical Dx based on the presence of hypomania and at least one depressive episode.

Tx/Mgmt: Same as bipolar type I (see above). Requires long-term treatment.

F. Cyclothymic Disorder

Buzz Words: Many periods of mild depression + hypomania for 2 years (without >2 months symptoms free)

Clinical Presentation: Age: 15–25 years

Gender: Female = male

Site of care: Outpatient

Chief Complaint: Complaints of frequent mood swings.

PMH/PSuH/PFH/PSoH: Associated with borderline personality disorder. Genetic predisposition likely given increased prevalence in families with major depression, bipolar disorder, and cyclothymia.

PPx: None

MoD: Unknown, multifactorial

Dx:

1. Rule out substance use.
2. This is a difficult Dx and essentially a Dx of exclusion if the patient has had over 2 years of symptoms ranging from depression to hypomania. Follow same steps as bipolar disorder type 1.

Tx/Mgmt: Same as bipolar disorder (see above). This is a chronic disorder and one-third of patients are eventually diagnosed with bipolar disorder.

Anxiety Disorders

A. Generalized Anxiety Disorders
Buzz Words: Excessive/uncontrollable worry (about many things!) + >6 months + adverse effect on function (missing work, not doing well in school, etc.)

Clinical Presentation: Age: Early 20s

Gender: 2:1, female:male

Site of care: Outpatient

Chief Complaint: Patient may present with non-psychiatric complaint such as insomnia, headaches, chest pain/palpitations, shortness of breath whereas others main complaint can be persistent daily anxiety.

PMH/PSuH/PFH/PSoH: Past medical history of MDD, phobias, or PD increase likelihood of Dx.

PPx: None, but avoiding caffeine and nicotine may decrease onset of anxiety.

MoD: Unknown etiology but biological and psychosocial factors seem to play a role. Neural evidence suggests a disruption in the connectivity of the amygdala and other areas of the brain that process fear and anxiety.

Dx: Considered a Dx of exclusion.
1. Evaluate for medical disorders (thyroid abnormalities and Cushing disease).
2. Inquire about substance use (alcohol, caffeine, nicotine, illicit substances).
3. Rule out PD (see below) and depression (see above).

Tx/Mgmt: Combination therapy is most effective: psychotherapy (cognitive behavior therapy [CBT]) and pharmacotherapy:
1. SSRIs, Buspirone, and Venlafaxine
2. If benzodiazepines (clonazepam, diazepam) are used, taper off soon given risk of tolerance and dependence.

B. Panic Disorder
Buzz Words: Unexpected debilitating intense fear (panic attack) + persistent fear of having attacks + change in behaviors to avoid attacks

Clinical Presentation: Age: Common during mid-20s, but may occur at any age

99 AR

Bipolar I, II, and Cyclothymia

QUICK TIPS

Buzzword for Rapid Cycling four or more episodes (major depressive episode, manic, hypomanic) within 1 year → rapid cycling bipolar disorder

QUICK TIPS

Panic attack symptoms include: tachypnea, tachycardia, chest pain, palpitation, diaphoresis, hot flashes, nausea, tremor, dizziness, fear of dying, and depersonalization.

Gender: 2–3× more common in females

Site of care: Outpatient

Chief Complaint: Concern regarding having panic attacks and/or report changes in behavior in order to avoid attacks

PMH/PSuH/PFH/PSoH: Family history of PD in a first-degree relative increases risk of developing PD (4–8×).

PPx: Avoid caffeine and nicotine as such may induce panic attacks.

MoD: Multifactorial:

- Neurochemical dysfunction suggests chemical imbalances in the limbic system (decreased serotonin and GABA with increased norepinephrine activity). Such dysfunction in turn sends signals to the amygdala initiating a "fight-or-flight" response to non-threatening situations.
- Specific genes have also been implicated with PD (but that is beyond the shelf's scope), just remember there is a genetic predisposition.

Dx:

1. Rule out medical conditions or medications/drug use (refer to table).
2. Assess for depression (SIGECAPS), phobia, OCD, and PTSD.
3. Be sure to elucidate whether patient is suffering from agoraphobia.

Medical conditions	Congestive heart failure, angina, myocardial infarction, thyrotoxicosis, temporal lobe epilepsy, multiple sclerosis, pheochromocytoma, carcinoid syndrome, chronic obstructive pulmonary disease
Medications/ drugs	Amphetamines, caffeine, nicotine, cocaine, hallucinogen intoxication, alcohol or opiate withdrawal

Tx/Mgmt:

1. CBT + pharmacotherapy (SSRI, SNRI, TCAs). Paroxetine and Sertraline have the best long-term effect (should be started at low dose and increased slowly).
2. Benzodiazepines may be effective during acute attacks but should only be used temporarily due to risk of tolerance and dependency.

3. Variable course but often chronic, relapses are common with medical discontinuation (treat for at least 8–12 months).

C. Obsessive-Compulsive Disorders

Buzz Words: Recurrent urges + response to urge with repeated behavior/mental acts that decrease anxiety + time consuming (>1 hour/day) + distressing (egodystonic) + interfere with daily functioning → OCD

Clinical Presentation: Age: Early childhood

Gender: Females = males

Site of care: Outpatient

Chief Complaint: May be non-psychiatric, such as skin rashes (due to frequent hand washing), or complaints of repeated acts (mental/behavioral) that are distressing.

PMH/PSuH/PFH/PSoH: Associated with MDD, eating disorders, and other anxiety disorders. OCD had also been associated with head injury, epilepsy, and basal ganglia disorders.

PPx: None

MoD: Multifactorial: Neurochemical role with abnormal regulation of serotonin, genetics given higher prevalence of OCD in first-degree relatives, and monozygotic twins and psychosocial given OCD may be triggered by a stressful life event.

Note that OCD patients have higher activity in the orbital cortex and caudate nucleus.

Dx:

1. Evaluate severity of obsession and compulsions.
2. Distinguish between distress versus no distress over behaviors.

Tx/Mgmt:

1. SSRI are first-line (clomipramine, fluoxetine, paroxetine, sertraline → higher doses often needed for full effect).
2. CBT is considered as effective as pharmacotherapy and has shown long-lasting benefit.
3. Combination of medication and therapy leads to best outcomes.

D. Posttraumatic Stress Disorder

Buzz Words: Prior witness of actual or threatened death/serious injury of self or others + re-experiencing (nightmares, flashbacks) + avoidance of trauma-related stimuli + increased arousal (trouble sleeping, irritability, hypervigilance) + >1 month duration.

QUICK TIPS

If patient is not distressed by obsession/compulsions (egosyntonic) → obsessive compulsive personality disorder

QUICK TIPS

Common Patterns of OCD
- Contamination → hand washing
- Doubt → checking
- Symmetry → taking a long time do perform tasks
- Intrusive thoughts → usually violent or sexual

Clinical Presentation: Age: Any age

Gender: Female > males

Site of care: Outpatient

Chief Complaint: Patients may report guilt, poor concentration, sleep disturbance, irritability, substance abuse, memory loss, depression, and suicidality.

PMH/PSuH/PFH/PSoH: Substance abuse and depression are frequent comorbidities.

PPx: None

MoD: (1) PTSD's fear conditioning occurs just as classical conditioning does. The patient comes to associate a stimulus (e.g., dark alleys) with a conditioned response (e.g., fear of alleys) in the absence of the unconditioned stimulus (e.g., rape). (2) Hippocampus and the amygdala are areas of the brain involved in fear learning.

Dx: This is a clinical Dx. Differentiate from phobias, OCD, or malingering (reporting symptoms with the purpose of secondary gain such as getting out of work, disability remuneration, etc.).

Tx/Mgmt:

1. Pharmacological: SSRIs, TCAs (imipramine, doxepin), MAOI, anticonvulsants (for flashbacks and nightmares).
2. Therapy: CBT, relaxation training, support groups, family therapy, and eye movement desensitization and reprocessing (EMDR).
3. Combination therapy is most effective.

Phobic Disorders (Specific and Social Phobias)

A. Specific Phobia

Buzz Words: Excessive fear of a specific object/situation (animal, blood, heights, flying) + recognition that fear is unreasonable + avoidance + interference with daily life

Clinical Presentation: Age: Early childhood

Gender: Female > male

Site of care: Outpatient

Chief Complaint: Distress over fear and avoidance of situations or objects

PMH/PSuH/PFH/PSoH: History of traumatic experience

PPx: None

MoD: Multifactorial, with genetic and neurochemical factors playing a role in disease development. Patients have also been shown to have increased activation of the amygdala.

Dx:
1. Rule out medical conditions: thyroid studies (hypo/hyperthyroidism), fasting glucose (hypoglycemia), urine 5-hydroxyindoleacetic acid (if concerned about a pheochromocytoma).
2. Also perform a urine drug screen to rule out substance-induced anxiety.

Tx/Mgmt:
1. CBT with desensitization (graded exposure to triggered object/situation) is most effective treatment:
   - Pharmacological treatment has not been shown to be effective.

B. Social Phobia

Buzz Words: Fear of embarrassment or humiliation + avoidance of social situations + decreased functionality (turning down promotions, poor sleep, etc.) + onset during adolescence

Clinical Presentation: Age: Mid-teens

Gender: Female = male

Site of care: Outpatient

Chief Complaint: Debilitating anxiety regarding social situations

PMH/PSuH/PFH/PSoH: Shy temperament is a risk factor

PPx: None

MoD: Same as specific phobia (see above)

Dx: Same as specific phobia (see above)

Tx/Mgmt:
1. Paroxetine and Venlafaxine are the only two FDA-approved agents for social phobia.
2. Beta-blockers and benzodiazepines may be used for performance anxiety (chose beta-blocker over benzos due to less sedating effects), cognitive behavioral therapies are a helpful adjunct.

Substance Use Disorders

Although the DSM V has combined both substance abuse and substance dependence under the category of "substance use disorders," you may be asked to distinguish between the two. Here is the distinction between the different classifications.

Substance abuse disorder highlights the social repercussions of using a substance. These repercussions include:
- Failure to fulfill responsibilities at school/work/home
- Using substance in a hazardous situation (driving while drunk)

- Continuous use despite these problems for over 1 year

Substance dependence disorder on the other hand, highlights physiological symptoms. These symptoms include:

- Tolerance (having to use larger amounts of the substance for the same effect)
- Withdrawal (having symptoms when not using the substance)
- Failed attempts to decrease use
- Spending significant time attempting to obtain substance
- Isolation from other aspects of life (work, school, relationships)
- Taking larger amounts of the substance than intended

Symptoms of Substance Intoxication and Withdrawal

Drug	Intoxication	Withdrawal
Tobacco/ nicotine	Insomnia, restlessness, anxiety, nausea	Irritability, headache, anxiety, weight gain, difficulty concentrating
Alcohol	Disinhibited behavior, mood changes, talkativeness, unsteady on feet	Tremors, hallucinations and/ or delusions, tachycardia, hypertension; life-threatening.
Opiates	Pupillary constriction, drowsiness, slurred speech	Abdominal pain and diarrhea, muscle ache, rhinorrhea, lacrimation, dilated pupils, piloerection
Cannabis	Increased appetite, dry mouth, conjunctival injection, impaired judgment, euphoria/ anxiety, paranoia	None

Drug	Intoxication	Withdrawal
Phencyclidine (PCP)	Psychosis, violence, impulsiveness, agitation, delirium, nystagmus	Sudden onset of intoxication symptoms without recurrent drug use
Cocaine	Tactile hallucinations, insomnia, confusion, elevated mood	Depression, malaise, increased appetite, nightmares
Benzodiazepines	Drowsiness, respiratory depression; increased potency with alcohol	Rebound anxiety, seizure, tremor, tachycardia, hypertension; life-threatening

Suicidal Identification

In the topic of suicidality, the family medicine shelf will most likely ask you to identify risk factors associated with suicide as well as the immediate triage and treatment for a suicidal individual.

Use the mnemonic SAD PERSONS to gauge risk factors for suicide:

- Sex (male>female)
- Age (older)
- Depression
- Previous attempt
- Ethanol/substance abuse
- Rational thought (can articulate plan)
- Sickness (suffers from chronic illness)
- Organized plan/access to weapon
- No spouse (single/divorced/widowed)
- Social support (lack of)

You should assess the following:

- Does the person have thoughts related to dying or committing suicide?
- Is there a plan? (i.e., buy pills and take them at midnight.)
- Does he or she have means to carry out a plan? (i.e., patient can get pills from family member.)
- Any previous attempts?

If patient is found to be acutely suicidal, hospitalization at an inpatient unit is required (even if this goes against a patient's will).

MNEMONIC

Use the CAGE questionnaire to assess for alcohol related issues:
1. Have you tried to Cut down your drinking?
2. Have you ever been Annoyed by others asking about your drinking?
3. Do you ever feel Guilty about drinking?
4. Have you ever had to have a drink first thing in the morning (Eye-opener)?

QUICK TIPS

Females are more likely to attempt suicide, but males are more likely to succeed in their attempt

QUICK TIPS

Prior suicide attempt is the most predictive risk factor for additional attempts.

GUNNER PRACTICE

1. A 40-year-old woman presents for a follow up appointment. She reports increased sweating, palpitations, and weight loss for the past 8 months. She also reports that her family dog passed away 2 weeks ago, which has been hard on the family. She works as a social worker at a local clinic and has been missing work more often due to being worried about everything. Her husband reports that his wife spends a lot of time worrying about their children when they are in daycare, though they have never gotten called for any issues. She worries about family finances despite her husband reassurance as well as her sister's health, who has no medical problems. Which of the following is the most likely diagnosis?
   A. Thyroid pathology
   B. Adjustment disorder
   C. Generalized anxiety disorder
   D. Obsession compulsive disorder
   E. Social anxiety
   F. Panic disorder with agoraphobia

2. A 21-year-old college student comes to the office for a checkup after he developed acute onset of diarrhea and abdominal pain yesterday. He also reports acute onset of rhinorrhea during the past 2 days but denies any fevers, coughing, or sick contacts despite living in a dorm. When asked about classes he looks nervous and says that he would rather not talk about it. He reports having wisdom teeth surgery 2 months ago and being prescribed Percocet for pain management. He does not report changes in his diet. His social history is significant for intermittent use of marijuana and alcohol on the weekends. Physical exam is significant for clear rhinorrhea without any turbinate or septum erythema and soft abdomen with mild tenderness to palpation throughout. What is the most likely reason for this patient's symptoms?
   A. Gastroenteritis
   B. Common cold
   C. Cocaine withdrawal
   D. Marijuana withdrawal
   E. Opiate withdrawal

3. A 50-year-old male recently diagnosed with prostate cancer presents as a new patient to your office. He reports that since receiving the diagnosis 3 weeks ago, he has felt more fatigued than usual. He reports decreased appetite but has not had any weight loss.

He also reports feeling extremely guilty about neglecting his health and continues to blame himself about his recent diagnosis. Though he usually enjoys playing chess with friends, he has not gone to chess club for the past 2 weeks because "he doesn't feel like it." He has been unable to sleep as well as he usually does. Since the diagnosis he has also had trouble coming up with lesson plans for his 7th grade class and missed 2 days of school last week. What is the most likely diagnosis?

A. Adjustment disorder
B. Major depressive disorder
C. Dysthymic disorder
D. Cyclothymic disorder
E. Primary insomnia

ANSWERS: What Would Gunner Jess/Jim Do?

1. WWGJD? A 40-year-old woman presents for a follow up appointment. She reports increased sweating, palpitations, and weight loss for the past 8 months. She also reports that her family dog passed away 2 weeks ago, which has been hard on the family. She works as a social worker at a local clinic and has been missing work more often due to being worried about everything. Her husband reports that his wife spends a lot of time worrying about their children when they are in daycare, though they have never gotten called for any issues. She worries about family finances despite her husband reassurance as well as her sister's health, though she has no medical problems. Physical exam is completely unremarkable and lab results show normal hemoglobin and thyroid panel. Which of the following is the most likely diagnosis?

Answer: C, Generalized anxiety disorder

Explanation: This patient has been experiencing anxiety over multiple areas of her life, including her finances, children, family members without any particular explanation (family is stable financially, children and sister are healthy and well). Hence, her diagnosis is most consistent with generalized anxiety disorder. Her anxiety has become debilitating to the point that she is missing work. This is important to note that she is missing work because of worrying about things and not because she has a fear of being embarrassed at work (E) or fear of public places and not being able to escape (F). Though she does have some physiologic symptoms that are associated with hyperthyroidism, her exam and lab work are not consistent with thyroid pathology.

A. Thyroid pathology → Incorrect. Although hyperthyroidism could be considered in this case given the patient's increased sweating, palpitations, and weight loss, the cluster of anxiety-related symptoms makes this diagnosis less likely.

B. Adjustment disorder → Incorrect. Although the family pet passed away and may have been a stressful moment for the family, such occurrence does not explain the generalized worries.

D. Obsession compulsive disorder → Incorrect. Patient does not report any history of obsessions or behavioral/mental compulsions that aid with decreasing anxiety.

E. Social anxiety → Incorrect. No evidence of fear of being embarrassed or symptoms being brought on by having to do something in front of others.

F. Panic disorder with agoraphobia → Incorrect. Though patient has avoided work, she has no history of panic attacks or evidence that her missing work is a product of being scared of being in public places.

2. WWGJD? A 21-year-old college student comes to the office for a check up after he developed acute onset of diarrhea and abdominal pain yesterday. He also reports acute onset of rhinorrhea during the past 2 days but denies any fevers, coughing, or sick contacts despite living in a dorm. When asked about classes, he looks nervous and says that he would rather not talk about it. He reports having wisdom teeth surgery 2 months ago and being prescribed Percocet for pain management. He does not report changes in his diet. His social history is significant for intermittent use of marijuana and alcohol on the weekends. Physical exam is significant for clear rhinorrhea without any turbinate or septum erythema and soft abdomen with mild tenderness to palpation throughout. What is the most likely reason for this patient's symptoms?

Answer: E, Opiate withdrawal

Explanation: This question challenges you to think about substance intoxication and withdrawal symptoms in a young patient. As you read the vignette, you should note a few red flags, including not wanting to talk about school, access to pain mediation, and substance use. Given the acute onset of abdominal pain and rhinorrhea on exam, the patient is most likely suffering from opiate withdrawal.

A. Gastroenteritis → Incorrect. Although acute onset of diarrhea could be due to viral or bacterial illness, lack of recent diet changes or sick contacts makes this diagnosis unlikely.

B. Common cold → Incorrect. Also a possible diagnosis given acute onset of rhinorrhea and some abdominal pain; however, lack of fevers, coughing, or sick contacts and recent prescription of opiates makes this less likely.

C. Cocaine withdrawal → Incorrect. Unlikely given cocaine withdrawal is often characterized by rebound anxiety and depression as well as headaches and tremulousness. Physical exam also does not seem consistent with cocaine use given normal appearance of nasal cavity.

D. Marijuana withdrawal → Incorrect. Withdrawal symptoms are not seen with cannabis discontinuation.

3. WWGJD? A 50-year-old male recently diagnosed with prostate **cancer** presents as a new patient to your office. He reports that since receiving the diagnosis **3 weeks ago,** he has felt more **fatigued** than usual. He reports **decreased appetite** but has not had any weight loss. He also reports feeling extremely **guilty about neglecting his health** and continues to blame himself about his recent diagnosis. Though he usually enjoys playing chess with friends, he **has not gone to chess club** for the past 2 weeks because **"he doesn't feel like it."** He has been **unable to sleep** as well as he usually does. Since the diagnosis he has also had **trouble coming up with lesson plans** for his seventh grade class and **missed 2 days** of school last week. What is the most likely diagnosis?

Answer: B, Major depressive disorder

Explanation: This is a classic question stem for major depressive disorder. As you go through the case, make a note, length of symptoms, whether the patient has sad mood or anhedonia, and then count the SIGECAPS symptoms presented. This patient has been experiencing symptoms for 3 weeks, shows anhedonia by not wanting to go play chess, and has had sleep disturbance, guilt, decreased appetite, impaired functioning. His constellation of symptoms is consistent with a diagnosis of major depressive disorder.

A. Adjustment disorder → Incorrect. Although the cancer diagnosis may have increased distress on the patient's life, emotional behavioral symptoms that are out of proportion to intensity of stressor his constellation of symptoms.

C. Dysthymic disorder → Incorrect. This diagnosis is not correct due to both time frame and severity of symptoms. First, dysthymia is diagnosis once symptoms have been present for at least 2 years. Secondly, dysthymic symptoms often do not impair daily functioning. Given this patient has had symptoms for 3 weeks and has had impairment of his daily functioning, this diagnosis is incorrect.

D. Cyclothymic disorder → Incorrect. Given patient has no history of hypomania or any manic symptoms (DIG FAST) this diagnosis is incorrect.

E. Primary insomnia → Incorrect. Though this patient reports difficulty sleeping and may have a concomitant diagnosis of insomnia, his constellation of symptoms are most consistent with MDD.

Diseases of the Nervous System and Special Senses

Jacob Cox, Leo Wang, Hao-Hua Wu, and Katherine Margo

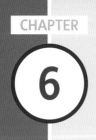

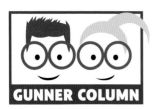

GUNNER COLUMN

Introduction

Diseases of the nervous system and special senses oftentimes have a dramatic impact on patients' quality of life or even survival. Moreover, their assessment and management often involves complex anatomic and pathophysiologic concepts. As such, these diseases are often tested extensively on standardized exams.

The nervous system refers to the brain, spinal cord, sensory organs, and all of the nerves that connect these organs with the rest of the body. Obviously, this plays a critical role in virtually every aspect of life and is intimately intertwined with all of the other organ systems. Dysfunction in the nervous system can result in pain, disability, and death. Similarly, the special senses refer to the senses that have a specialized organ or organ system devoted to them (e.g., vision, hearing, balance, smell, and taste). These are essential to our ability to interact with the world around us. So while special sense disorders are rarely life threatening, they are often debilitating and severely impact one's quality of life.

This chapter addresses a wide array of the most common and the most severe diseases of the nervous system and special senses. They are categorized as infectious, neoplasms, cerebrovascular, spinal, cranial, peripheral, pain-related, movement, paroxysmal, traumatic, mechanical, or congenital. All sections are high-yield, but cerebrovascular, movement, and ophthalmic disorders are particularly high-yield. You should also become comfortable with the nervous system's unique vocabulary terms and basic concepts regarding the circulation and pathways.

Only about 1%–5% of the NBME Family Medicine shelf will focus on disease of the nervous system. These questions generally cover fundamental concepts and treatment plans, rather than delving into nuanced specifics. As such, be sure to familiarize yourself with the presentation of various diseases and the appropriate diagnostic and therapeutic steps, but don't stress knowing every minor detail!

Cerebrovascular Disease

Transient Ischemic Attack

Buzz Words: Loss of speech + weakness + no findings on magnetic resonance imaging (MRI)

Clinical Presentation: Often a warning sign of progressing formation of a thrombus or formation of small emboli. Patients often present with stroke symptoms for only 10–60 minutes and therefore are not symptomatic once reaching a treatment center, which may delay diagnosis.

PPx: (1) Treat hypertension, (2) statins to treat hyperlipidemia, (3) aspirin, (4) treat diabetes

MoD: (1) Thrombotic (clot forming at site of infarction), (2) hypoxic (secondary to hypoxemia or hypoperfusion), (3) embolic (embolus from distal site travels to brain vasculature)

Dx:

1. Non-contrast head CT to rule out hemorrhage
2. Brain MRI to look for ischemic lesions
3. Carotid duplex scan or computed tomography (CT) angiogram of head/neck to look for extracranial stenosis
4. Cardiac echo to look for thrombus in left atrium (e.g., in patients with atrial fibrillation)

Tx/Mgmt:

1. Aspirin
2. Clopidogrel
3. Warfarin

Stroke

Buzz Words: Sudden onset of neurologic change or focal paralysis (specific symptoms in Tables 6.1 and 6.2)

Clinical Presentation: Often elderly patient (peak age: 80–84), more common in men than women; smoking is a risk factor; OCPs are risk factor. Symptoms vary depending on location of stroke.

Lacunar stroke syndrome may also occur in pts w/chronic HTN or DM who then develop infarction in territories of deep penetrating arteries 2/2 arteriolosclerosis. Five classic lacunar stroke syndromes are shown in Table 6.2.

PPx: (1)Treat hypertension, (2) statins to treat hyperlipidemia, (3) aspirin, (4) treat diabetes, (5) ultrasound duplex is NOT recommended in asymptomatic patients.

MoD: Sudden reduction in supply of blood to brain tissue:

- Ischemic (70%–80%; from blockage of blood flow)

TABLE 6.1 Location of Stroke Correlated With Symptoms

Location of Stroke	Symptoms
Middle cerebral artery (MCA) (90% of cases)	• Contralateral hemiparesis and sensory loss in the face and upper extremity • Expressive aphasia • If Broca's area involved in the dominant (left) hemisphere • Visual field defects • Head and eyes deviate toward the side of the lesion
Anterior cerebral artery (ACA)	• Contralateral hemiparesis and sensory loss in the lower extremity • ACA stroke: contralateral paresis/sensory loss in lower extremity
Posterior cerebral artery (PCA)	• Ipsilateral sensory loss of the face, ninth, and tenth cranial nerves • Contralateral sensory loss of the limbs • Limb ataxia
Vertebrobasilar artery system	• Vertigo, ataxia • Ipsilateral sensory loss in face • Contralateral hemiparesis and sensory loss in the trunk and limbs

TABLE 6.2 Lacunar Stroke Locations and Symptoms

Lacunar Stroke Syndrome	Symptoms
Pure motor stroke	• Weakness of the face, arm, and leg on one side of the body • Absent sensory or cortical signs (aphasia, neglect, apraxia, hemianopsia) • Most common, about 50% of lacunar strokes
Pure sensory stroke	• Sensory defect (numbness) of the face, arm, and leg on one side of the body • Absent motor or cortical signs
Ataxic hemiparesis syndrome	• Ipsilateral weakness and limb ataxia out of proportion to the motor defect, possible gait deviation to the affected side • Absent cortical signs
Dysarthria-clumsy hand syndrome	• Facial weakness, dysarthria, dysphagia, and slight weakness, and clumsiness of one hand • Absent sensory or cortical signs • Least common
Mixed sensorimotor stroke	• Hemiparesis of hemiplegia with sensory abnormality on the same side

- Atherosclerotic → most common type
- Embolic → from carotid stenosis, Afib, valvular heart disease, deep vein thrombosis reaching brain via patent foramen ovale (PFO)
- Hemorrhagic (20%–30%; from bleeding)

Dx:
1. Non-contrast head CT to rule out hemorrhage
2. Brain MRI to look for ischemic lesions
3. Carotid duplex scan or CT angiogram of head/neck to look for extracranial stenosis
4. Cardiac echo to look for thrombus in left atrium (e.g., in patients with atrial fibrillation)

Tx/Mgmt: Varies depending on type of stroke. Unlikely to be tested since these are inpatient treatments.

Subclavian Steal Syndrome

Buzz Words: Claudication of arm (coldness, tingling, muscle pain) + visual symptoms + equilibrium problems (posterior neurologic signs) + symptoms in s/o arm exercise

Clinical Presentation: Subclavian steal syndrome is a phenomenon whereby an arteriosclerotic stenotic plaque at the origin of the subclavian (before the takeoff of the vertebral) does not allow enough blood supply to reach the arm for normal activity; therefore the blood pressure would be low on the affected arm. After doing the exercise of the affected arm, the blood flow can be stolen from the ipsilateral vertebral artery (retrograde flow) in order to supply the blood into the brachial artery. As a result, there is not enough blood flow going into the posterior circulation that will supply the brain stem.

PPx: N/A

MoD: Significant stenosis/occlusion proximal to origin subclavian artery → lower pressure in distal subclavian artery → blood flows from contralateral vertebral artery to basilar artery → flow reversal may occur in blood flow of ipsilateral vertebral artery, away from brainstem → usually asymptomatic, but may lead to arm ischemia or vertebrobasilar ischemia.

Dx:
1. Blood pressure (difference in brachial systolic BP of >15 mm Hg)
2. Ultrasound duplex scan
2. Arteriogram (to show reversal of flow of the affected vertebral artery)

Tx/Mgmt: Bypass surgery

Vascular Dementia

Buzz Words: Stepwise decline of cognitive function; memory loss + over the course of disease with history of multiple ischemic or hemorrhagic strokes (weakness, dizziness)

Clinical Presentation: This is often tested in the setting of memory loss as opposed to stroke symptoms.

PPx: (1) Measures that reduce atherosclerotic disease (e.g., control HTN, DM, HLD)

MoD: A variety of vascular factors including multiple cerebral infarctions that occur over time.

Dx:
1. CT
2. MRI

Tx/Mgmt: Address risk factors for vascular disease risk factors.

Headache

HEADACHE MANAGEMENT

Type	Tension Headache	Migraine	Cluster Headache
Presentation	• Bilateral "bandlike" pressure • Lasts 4–6 h • Normal physical exam	• ± Aura, photophobia • Related to food/emotions/menses • Rare: aphasia, numbness, dysarthria	• Episodic pain • Unilateral periorbital intense pain • Lacrimation • Eye reddening • Nasal stuffiness • Lid ptosis
Treatment	• NSAIDs • Acetaminophen	• Avoid triggers • NSAIDs • Triptans (5-HT1 agonists)	• Sumitriptan • Octreotide • Oxygen
Prophylaxis		If three attacks per month: • Propranolol • Sodium valproate • Topiramate • Others	• Verapamil • Prednisone • Sodium valproate

NSAIDs, Nonsteroidal anti-inflammatory drugs.

Migraine

Buzz Words: Aura + N/V + phonophobia + photophobia

Clinical Presentation: More common in women. Pain often exacerbated by activity. Unilateral, pulsating pain. Twenty-five percent of patients have visual/auditory/somatosensory/motor aura (focal neurologic symptoms ≤1 hour before headache). Most common auras are "scintillating scotomas" (perception of bright or flashing lights) or visual field defects. Often associated w/ photophobia, phonophobia, N/V.

Common triggers include fluctuations in estrogen, OCPs, food containing tyramine or nitrates/nitrites (e.g., chocolate, wine, cheese, processed meats, aged foods).

PPx: (1) Avoid trigger, such as foods containing tyramine

MoD: Previously popular theory related to dilatation of blood vessels, but this is no longer supported. Likely involves neuronal dysfunction leading to various intra- and extracranial changes that induce migraine.

Dx: Clinical

Tx/Mgmt: Acute treatment:
1. Avoid triggers
2. NSAIDs → first-line; if fails, try another NSAID before escalating
3. Sumatriptan → if NSAIDs fail

Preventative treatment:
1. Beta-blockers → if frequent/severe migraines or if failed abortive Tx's
2. Calcium-channel blockers → if beta-blockers contraindicated
3. Amitriptyline → beware side effects
4. Topiramate → contraindicated in pregnancy (teratogenic)

Tension Headache

Buzz Words: Young woman with bilateral and band-like pain + localized to frontal or occipital regions

Clinical Presentation: Most common form of headache by far. More common in women. Pain is bilateral and band-like pain, localized to frontal or occipital regions, and may involve neck. It is associated with stress and fatigue with a duration of >30 minutes; no aura, photophobia, phonophobia, or nausea/vomiting.

PPx: (1) Avoid stressful situations

MoD: Most common headache in adults. Cause is likely multifactorial, but precise mechanism is unknown. Environmental and genetic factors appear contributory.

Dx: Clinical. No tests required. Clinical picture is sufficient. However, you should exclude:
1. Migraine: Usu. no physical findings, but rare cases → aphasia, numbness, dysarthria, or weakness
2. Cluster headache: red, tearing eye with rhinorrhea, Horner syndrome
3. Giant cell arteritis: visual loss, tenderness of the temporal area
4. Pseudotumor cerebri: papilledema + diplopia from central nerve (CN) VI palsy

Tx/Mgmt: Acute treatment:
1. Relaxation (avoid high-stress situations, try hot baths, massage, biofeedback)
2. NSAIDs (shorten duration and intensity)
   a. Caffeine ($\uparrow$ efficacy of NSAIDs and acetaminophen; reserve for patients who fail simple analgesics)
3. Acetaminophen
   Preventative treatment:
1. Amitriptyline (if frequent/severe; $\downarrow$ duration and intensity by 50% if taken prophylactically; beware narrow therapeutic window)

Cluster Headache

Buzz Words: Unilateral periorbital headache + stabbing pain in man + lacrimation

Clinical Presentation: It is more common in men. Unilateral periorbital headache occurs with stabbing pain, often with ipsilateral autonomic symptoms (tearing, conjunctival injection, nasal congestion, rhinorrhea, ptosis, miosis, diaphoresis). Precipitated by EtOH (often within 1 hour of use). Repetitive attacks in clusters, usually during same time of day or same season of year.

PPx: N/A

MoD: Cause is likely complex and not completely known. May involve hypothalamic activation with secondary activation of trigeminal-autonomic reflex.

Dx:
1. Clinical criteria (fulfill all of the following):
   a. More than five attacks
   b. Severe unilateral orbital, supraorbital, and/or temporal pain more than 15 minutes
   c. One of following: restlessness, agitation, miosis, ptosis, ear fullness, eyelid edema, facial swelling/flushing, conjunctival injection/lacrimation, nasal congestion/rhinorrhea

Tx/Mgmt:
1. High-flow 100% O_2 (12–15 L/min via nonrebreather mask w/pt seated upright)
2. Sumatriptan (contraindicated in cardiovascular disease, stroke, uncontrolled HTN, or pregnancy)
3. Ergots (limited evidence, not first-line)

Pseudotumor Cerebri (aka Idiopathic Intracranial Hypertension)

Buzz Words: Young overweight woman taking retionids or vitamin A derivatives for skin conditions presenting with headaches

Clinical Presentation: Daily pulsatile headaches are worsened by eye movement, diplopia, blurry vision (2/2 papilledema). NO focal neurologic signs or mental status changes. Worst complication is vision loss.

PPx: (1) Avoidance of excessive vitamin A intake, (2) weight loss

↓ Cerebrospinal fluid (CSF) resorption in arachnoid granulations → ↑ intracranial pressure (ICP). Equilibrium is ultimately achieved between CSF inflow and outflow, but this occurs at higher ICP than normal. Most commonly seen in obese females of childbearing age.

Dx:
1. Fundoscopic exam (may see papilledema)
2. MRI/CT → flattening of the posterior globe (100% positive predictive value); r/o central venous thrombosis or tumor or other CSF-obstructing lesion
3. Lumbar puncture will show elevated CSF pressure

Tx/Mgmt:
1. **Lifestyle changes:** Discontinue inciting agents (e.g., excess vitamin A, long-term tetracyclines); weight loss in obese pts.
2. **Medical:** Carbonic anhydrase inhibitor (e.g., mannitol) or systemic corticosteroids if visual disturbances (lowers CSF pressure).
3. **Procedural:** Serial lumbar punctures.
4. **Surgical:** Lumboperitoneal shunt; optic nerve sheath fenestration.

Mild Traumatic Brain Injury (Concussion)

Buzz Words: Football player + boxer + acute loss of consciousness + acute ΔMS, inability to recall incident + headache

Clinical Presentation: Transient loss of conscious, confusion, or amnesia associated with blunt trauma to head.

PPx: (1) Avoidance of activities that raise risk for head trauma, (2) wearing a helmet during activities like cycling, skateboarding, etc.

MoD: Exact mechanism unknown

Dx: Neurological assessment (including c-spine)

Tx/Mgmt: Rest and avoidance of activity where injury may be repeated (duration of rest is source of controversy).

Dementia

Alzheimer Disease

Buzz Words: Older individual + progressive forgetfulness + chronic and progressive + <24 on mini-mental state examination (MMSE) + apraxia + aphasia + agnosia + impairs ADLs (vs. mild cognitive impairment or normal aging)

Clinical Presentation: Patients with Alzheimer disease are typically older than 60 years and present with reduction in short-term memory (unable to remember newly learned facts) and word-finding difficulty. Paranoia, personality changes, and executive dysfunction may also be prominent. Women have 3× increased prevalence compared to men. If Down syndrome in past medical history, symptoms will present much earlier in lifespan.

PPx: None

MoD: Mediated by amyloid beta plaques (extracellular) and neurofibrillary tangles (intracellular)

Dx:

1. MMSE
2. Rule out reversible causes of dementia by looking at TSH, T3, T4 or B12 levels, RPR for syphilis
3. Head MRI to r/o structural lesions, will show diffuse atrophy/enlarged ventricles with disproportionate atrophy of the hippocampus

Tx/Mgmt:

1. Donepezil (acetylcholinesterase inhibitor)
2. Galantamine, rivastigmine (AChE inhibitors)
3. For moderate or severe → Memantine (NMDA antagonist):
   - Antipsychotics, such as Olanzapine and quetiapine, are sometimes used to control psychosis, aggression, and agitation that may develop.

Frontotemporal Dementia (Pick Disease)

Buzz Words: Inappropriate behavior/poor judgment + personality changes + disinhibition + hypersexuality + snout reflex

Clinical Presentation: Frontal temporal dementia (FTLD) is the second most common cause of early onset dementia (after Alzheimer). On the shelf, it is can be identified as a patient with memory difficulties who is disinhibited (e.g., says things that are uncharacteristically offensive). It presents in patients older than 55 years with the chief complaint being one of two variants: behavioral and languages.

PPx: None

MoD: Severe atrophy of the frontal and temporal lobes secondary

Dx:

1. MMSE, neurobehavioral assessment
2. CT/MRI → show disproportionate atrophy of frontal/temporal lobes
3. Rule out reversible dementia (thyroid, B12)

Tx/Mgmt: Only symptomatic treatment is currently available (no FDA-approved drug):
- Olanzapine/antipsychotic for severe disinhibition, aggression, and agitation

Lewy Body Dementia

Buzz Words: Lilliputian hallucinations (benign hallucinations) + episodic confusion +impaired visuospatial function + dementia less than 12 months after onset of bradykinesia, tremor, abnormal posture, rigidity:
- If more than 12 months, Parkinson's disease with dementia (see below)

Clinical Presentation: Lewy body dementia (LBD) is high-yield because of its distinct Buzz Words in the setting of memory loss (e.g., Lilliputian hallucinations). If dementia more than 12 months, Parkinson's disease with dementia (see below). Patients present with parkinsonian symptoms (bradykinesia, tremor, abnormal posture, rigidity) and dementia (dementia may precede or follow parkinsonian symptoms).
- Visual hallucinations and **REM sleep behavior** disorders often seen.

PPx: None

MoD: Intra-cytoplasmic alpha-synuclein inclusions diffusely seen throughout the cortex and substantia nigra; they lead to degeneration of dopamine releasing neurons.

Dx: Clinical exam and history demonstrating parkinsonian syndrome, recurrent hallucinations, REM sleep behavior disorders, and dementia

Tx/Mgmt:
1. Treat parkinsonian features with levo-carbidopa (but may lead to worsening hallucinations/delirium)
2. Treat cognitive symptoms with acetylcholinesterase inhibitors (Donepezil)

Parkinson Disease

Buzz Words: Cogwheel rigidity + resting tremor + shuffling gait + akinesia + dementia after 12 months of symptom onset

Clinical Presentation: Parkinson disease (PD) is the second most common neurodegenerative disease (after Alzheimer) and is caused by the deposition of alpha-synuclein in the pigmented nuclei of the brainstem. The shelf exam will test your ability to recognize the diagnostic features of PD and the available therapies. In addition, PD patients sometimes develop dementia, and some patients with parkinsonian symptoms develop dementia very early in

QUICK TIPS

If a patient has hallucinations/paranoid delusions/episodic confusion early in the disease course, think Lewy body dementia. These are NOT common early in Alzheimer/FTLD.

their disease course. These patients will have more widespread alpha-synuclein deposition and diagnosed with LBD. PD can also be considered a **hypo**kinetic movement disorder.

The chief complaint will likely be one of four complaints: bradykinesia, resting tremor, postural instability, cogwheel rigidity. There is a possible link to repeated head trauma and organophosphate exposure may increase risk (toxic to dopaminergic substantia nigra neurons).

PPx: None

MoD: Loss of dopaminergic neurons in the basal ganglia and substantia nigra pars compacta with alpha-synuclein inclusions

Dx:

1. Clinical exam demonstrating tetrad of parkinsonian features
2. MRI/CT to rule out mimics of PD

Tx/Mgmt: Treatment cannot reverse the alpha-synuclein pathology, but focuses on symptom management.

1. Levo-carbidopa (carbidopa does not enter the central nervous system [CNS] and blocks degradation of L-dopa outside CNS)
2. Dopamine agonists (bromocriptine), less potent than L-dopa
3. Deep brain stimulation if L-dopa fails

Miscellaneous Neurologic Disorders

Essential Tremor

Buzz Words: Tremor that gets worse with movement

Clinical Presentation: High-frequency tremor with variable amplitude present at both rest and during intentional movements. Usually most prominent in hands. Often disrupts manual skills such as handwriting. Worse with caffeine.

PPx: N/A

MoD: Pathophysiology unknown.

Dx: Clinical. Tremor at rest and exertion. Improved with alcohol. Tremor should improve when patient is distracted from his or her movements.

Tx/Mgmt:

1. Propranolol
2. Primidone
3. Alcohol
4. Benzodiazepines (e.g., alprazolam, clonazepam)

Bell's Palsy (CN VII)

Buzz Words: Unlike stroke, forehead is also paralyzed.

Clinical Presentation: Paralysis of entire side of face. (NOTE: stroke paralyzes only lower half of the face.) Difficulty closing the eye, hyperacusis (sounds are extra loud because CN VII supplies stapedius muscle, which is a "shock absorber" on the ossicles), taste disturbances (b/c CN VII nerve provides taste to ⅔ of tongue).

PPx: N/A

MoD: Most cases = idiopathic. Some ½ Lyme disease, sarcoidosis, herpes zoster reactivation

Dx: Clinical exam: If patient CAN wrinkle forehead on affected side → worry about stroke. If patient CANNOT wrinkle forehead on affected side → Bell's palsy.

Tx/Mgmt:
1. Majority self-limited
2. Prednisone
3. Provide eye care (e.g., lubricant or suture lid closed temporarily)

Trigeminal Neuralgia

Buzz Words: "Knife stuck into face" + shooting pain + clusters of attacks

Clinical Presentation: Sharp burning/stabbing unilateral pain in CN V, distribution often precipitated by chewing, touching the face, or pronunciation of certain words (tongue strikes the back of front teeth). Patients describe the pain as feeling as if a knife is being stuck into the face. No neurologic deficits.

PPx: N/A

MoD: Some cases are idiopathic. Others are ½ compression of trigeminal nerve root.

Dx: There is no specific diagnostic test.

Tx/Mgmt:
1. Oxcarbazepine or carbamazepine = first-line
2. Aclofen and lamotragine = second-line
3. If refractory to medications → surgical decompression

Multiple Sclerosis

Buzz Words:
- Neurologic dysfunction separated in time and space (optic neuritis and internuclear opthalmoplegia, sensory loss, bladder dysfunction, trigeminal neuralgia, intention tremor) + young woman + Lhermitte's sign

Clinical Presentation: Multiple sclerosis (MS) is a demyelinating disease in which the CNS is demyelinated. It is named for the *multiple sclerosing plaques* of the white matter in the CNS. The symptoms can be relatively non-specific, although most patients present with symptoms

QUICK TIPS

Lhermitte's sign = electrical sensation down back and limbs when neck is flexed in the eye. It is unlikely you will be tested on the pathophysiology of multiple sclerosis on the shelf since this is not well understood. More likely, you will be tested on recognizing, diagnosing, and managing the disease. In this context, having an understanding of the breadth of knowledge of MS is important, especially the different clinical presentations that can affect how the disease presents over long periods of time.

PPx: None

MoD: Thought to be a contribution of environmental and genetic factors, related to early childhood virus infection → autoimmune destruction of oligodendrocytes, demyelination occurs in CNS only, thought to be related to vitamin D and T-cells reactive to myelin basic protein

Dx:

1. Clinical/neurological exam based on pattern of presentation
2. MRI: **white matter lesions that separate in space and time** (i.e., a lesion has to appear in two different places at two different times)
3. LP: CSF with oligoclonal bands

Tx/Mgmt:

1. Acute: steroids and plasmapheresis
2. Disease modifying: injectable medicines—IFN-1alpha, IFN-1beta, glatiramer (mimics myelin), natalizumab, ivoral medicines—fingolimod, teriflunomide, dimethyl fumarate
3. Physical therapy

Peripheral Neuropathies

	SPECIFIC PERIPHERAL NERVE NEUROPATHIES	
Nerve	**Precipitating Event Described in the Stem**	**Manifestations/ Presentation**
Ulnar	Biker, pressure on palms of hands, trauma to medial side of elbow	Wasting of hypothenar eminence, pain in fourth and fifth fingers
Radial	Pressure of inner, upper arm; falling asleep with arm over back of chair ("Saturday night palsy"); using crutches and pressure in the axilla	Wrist drop

Peripheral Neuropathies—cont'd

SPECIFIC PERIPHERAL NERVE NEUROPATHIES

Nerve	Precipitating Event Described in the Stem	Manifestations/ Presentation
Lateral cutaneous nerve of thigh—meralgia paresthetica	Obesity, pregnancy, sitting with crossed legs	Pain/numbness of outer aspect of one thigh
Tarsal tunnel (tibial nerve)	Worsens with walking	Pain/numbness in ankle and sole of foot
Peroneal	High boots, pressure on back of knee	Weak foot with decreased dorsiflexion and eversion
Median—carpal tunnel syndrome	Typist, carpenters, working with hands	Thenar wasting, pain/numbness in first three fingers

GUNNER PRACTICE

1. A 56-year-old woman comes in with a high frequency tremor of both hands. The tremors are mild at rest, but are exaggerated when she tries to make precise movements. She has noticed they are particularly prominent when she tries to cook, and recently dropped boiling water on herself due to the movements in her hands. She notices that this tremor tends to completely disappear when she consumes "sufficient alcohol." Which of the following is the most appropriate next step in management?
   A. Deep brain stimulation
   B. Alcohol
   C. Propanolol
   D. Psychiatric evaluation
   E. No treatment is indicated

ANSWERS: What Would Gunner Jess/Jim Do?

1. WWGJD? A 56-year-old woman comes in with a high-frequency tremor of both hands. The tremors are mild at rest, but are exaggerated when she tries to make precise movements. She has noticed they are particularly prominent when she tries to cook, and recently dropped boiling water on herself due to the movements in her hands. She notices that this tremor tends to completely disappear when she consumes "sufficient alcohol." Which of the following is the most appropriate next step in management?

Answer: C. Propanolol

Explanation: This is the first-line treatment for intention tremor, which is a tremor that gets worse with intentional movements and improves with alcohol.

A. Deep brain stimulation → Incorrect. This is a last resort treatment for intention tremor. Also helps PD tremor.

B. Alcohol → Incorrect. While this improves intention tremor, this cannot be prescribed pharmacologically.

D. Psychiatric evaluation → Incorrect. There is no psychiatric basis for tremors and this patient demonstrates no signs of psychiatric illness.

E. No treatment is indicated → Incorrect. This patient clearly is suffering and there are clear pharmacologic treatments for intention tremor.

Cardiovascular Disorders

Leo Wang, Junqian Zhang, Hao-Hua Wu, and
Katherine Margo

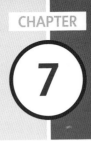

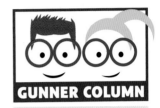

GUNNER COLUMN

The heart is one of the most dynamic organs in the human body. It provides driving force in the circulatory system and has the ability to adapt to a wide range of hemodynamic conditions. Dysfunction of the cardiovascular system can occur in many acute and chronic contexts and has both local and systemic manifestations. In this regard, cardiovascular disease is the **leading** cause of death in the United States, with a large number of these deaths being attributed to coronary artery disease.

On the family medicine shelf, this concept is important because the large numbers of these diseases are **preventable**. As such, the most important aspect within this chapter will be prophylaxis. Treatment will be particularly important for diseases that are risk factors for coronary artery disease and myocardial infarction—the big three here are hypertension, hyperlipidemia, and diabetes (discussed in endocrine). Focus on every aspect of these diseases as they are extremely important to manage considering they will eventually lead to infarction.

Coronary Artery Disease

Stable Angina

Buzz Words: Sub-sternal chest pressure or pain on EXERTION that goes away with rest

Clinical Presentation: Sub-sternal chest pressure or pain that may radiate to the arm, shoulder, neck, or jaw. Other features may include diaphoresis and shortness of breath:
- Note that women and the elderly may have atypical symptoms including epigastric pain
- No elevation in cardiac enzymes (troponin, creatine kinase)

Prophylactic (PPx): Preventable risk factors: (1) blood pressure control, (2) diet and exercise, (3) diabetes control, (4) smoking cessation, (5) cholesterol control

Mechanism of Disease (MoD): Chronic atherosclerotic disease of coronary vessels prevents adequate delivery of blood to the myocardium during periods of high oxygen demand.

Diagnostic Steps (Dx):

1. Baseline electrocardiogram (EKG)
2. Exercise EKG OR pharmacologic stress test OR exercise stress imaging:
   - Exercise EKG is only indicated if baseline EKG is normal
   - For patients with abnormal baseline EKG or who cannot tolerate exercise → pharmacologic stress (with coronary vasodilators—dipyridamole, regadenoson) echocardiography
3. Cardiac enzymes—no elevation in troponin or creatine kinase
4. Coronary angiogram:
   - Indicated in patients with abnormal non-invasive testing (i.e., EKG or echocardiogram)

Treatment/Management (Tx/Mgmt):

1. Treat modifiable risk factors—obesity, diabetes mellitus, cholesterol.
2. Sublingual nitroglycerin for acute exacerbations.
3. β-Blockers, calcium channel blockers (CCBs), or long-acting nitrates (isosorbide mononitrate) for chronic stable angina.

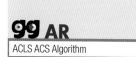

99 AR

ACLS ACS Algorithm

Unstable Angina

Buzz Words: Sub-sternal chest pressure or pain with exertion that occurs at rest

Clinical Presentation: Sub-sternal chest pressure or pain that may radiate to the arm, shoulder, neck, or jaw that is not necessarily related to exertion. Other features may include diaphoresis and shortness of breath:

- No elevation in cardiac enzymes (troponin, creatine kinase)

PPx: Preventable risk factors: (1) blood pressure control, (2) diet and exercise, (3) diabetes control, (4) smoking cessation, (5) cholesterol control

MoD: Atherosclerotic plaque instability that leads to temporary partial occlusion of coronary artery with subsequent resolution—note that the distinction between stable and unstable angina is based on clinical findings and not necessarily related to the degree of coronary occlusion.

Dx:

1. EKG—may show transient ST-segment depression during acute symptoms.
2. Exercise EKG OR pharmacologic stress test OR exercise stress imaging.
3. Cardiac enzymes—no elevation in troponin or creatine kinase.

Tx/Mgmt:
1. Immediate EMS care and hospital notification.
2. Sublingual nitroglycerin for acute symptoms.
3. Aspirin, β-blockers, heparin.
4. Coronary angiography ± angioplasty or CABG.

Non-ST-Elevation Myocardial Infarction

Buzz Words: ST-depressions in the setting of anginal chest pain ± radiation to the arm and jaw

Clinical Presentation: Non-ST-elevation myocardial infarction (NSTEMI): typical anginal chest pain (crushing substernal chest pressure is classic) ± radiation to jaw, shoulder, or arm ± diaphoresis, nausea, or vomiting

PPx: Control risk factors including atherosclerosis, hyperlipidemia, and diabetes mellitus (DM)

MoD: Acute plaque rupture within coronary circulation with partial occlusion or transient total occlusion that leads to partial-thickness myocardial infarction.

Dx:
1. EKG—ST-depressions in contiguous leads.
2. Cardiac enzymes—elevation of troponin and creatine kinase.

Tx/Mgmt:
1. Secondary prevention of future acute coronary syndrome with aspirin, β-blocker, ACE inhibitors or angiotensin receptor blockers (ARBs), statin, spironolactone:
   a. Avoid β-blockers in patients with bradycardia, decompensated heart failure with low ejection fraction, heart block, asthma, and chronic obstructive pulmonary disease (COPD)
   b. ARBs can be used in patients who are allergic to ACE inhibitors

MNEMONIC

OH BATMAN for the treatment of NSTEMI (oxygen, heparin, β-blockers, aspirin, thrombolysis, morphine, ACE inhibitors, nitroglycerine)

ST-Elevation Myocardial Infarction

Buzz Words: ST-elevation (Fig. 7.1) in contiguous leads in the setting of typical anginal chest pain (crushing substernal chest pressure is classic) ± radiation to jaw, shoulder, or arm ± diaphoresis, nausea, or vomiting

Clinical Presentation: Typical anginal chest pain (crushing substernal chest pressure is classic) ± radiation to jaw, shoulder, or arm ± diaphoresis, nausea, or vomiting. Ventricular arrhythmias are common after MI and are the most common cause of cardiac failure and death in the immediate post-MI period. Ventricular free-wall rupture, septal rupture, and papillary muscle rupture most

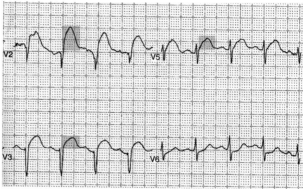

FIG. 7.1 ST-elevation myocardial infarction. Note the ST-elevations in contiguous leads V_1–V_4. (From https://en.wikipedia.org/wiki/Electrocardiography_in_myocardial_infarction.)

commonly occur during the first 7–10 days after MI. Posteromedial papillary muscle is most prone to rupture due to single blood supply from the right coronary artery. Ventricular aneurysms tend to occur months after MI.

PPx: Control risk factors including (1) atherosclerosis, (2) hyperlipidemia, and (3) DM

MoD: Acute plaque rupture within coronary circulation with complete occlusion leading to full-thickness myocardial infarction

Dx:

1. EKG—ST-elevations greater than 1 mm in contiguous leads
2. Cardiac enzymes—elevation of troponin and creatine kinase
   - Troponin is more sensitive but stays elevated for up to 2 weeks after MI → use CK-MB if suspicious for repeat-MI

Tx/Mgmt:

1. OH BATMAN—oxygen, heparin, β-blockers, aspirin, thrombolysis, morphine, ACE inhibitors, nitroglycerine:
   a. Give aspirin and typically heparin prior to coronary catheterization
2. Coronary catheterization (door-to-balloon time <90 minutes is ideal)
3. Secondary prevention of future acute coronary syndrome with aspirin, β-blocker, ACE inhibitors or ARBs, statin, spironolactone:
   a. Avoid β-blockers in patients with bradycardia, decompensated heart failure with low ejection fraction, heart block, asthma, and COPD
   b. ARBs can be used in patients who are allergic to ACE inhibitors (Fig. 7.2)

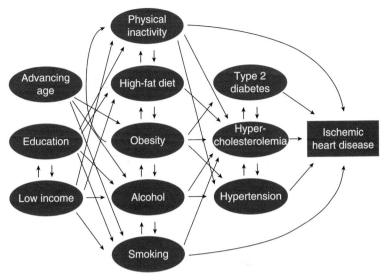

FIG. 7.2 Risk factors for MI.

Printzmetal Angina (Variant Angina)

Buzz Words: Young + female smokers with anginal chest pain, especially at night

Clinical Presentation: Young and middle-aged female smokers who present with typical chest pain, especially at night
- Associated with migraines and Raynaud phenomenon (i.e., other vasospasm-related disorders); can also occur secondary to cocaine use

PPx: Preventable risk factors: smoking, cocaine use

MoD: Coronary artery vasospasm leading to tissue ischemia/infarction

Dx:
1. EKG—typically normal but may show ST-segment abnormalities during episodes of vasospasm.
2. Coronary angiography with provocation testing with ergonovine or acetylcholine is the gold standard.

Tx/Mgmt:
1. CCBs or nitrates.
2. β-Blockers are contraindicated as they can lead to exacerbation of vasospasm (i.e., unopposed α-adrenergic stimulation).

Cardiac Arrhythmias

Atrial Fibrillation (Fig. 7.3)

Buzz Words: Irregularly irregular rhythm + absence of P-waves

MNEMONIC

CHA_2DS_2-VASc—Risk of Stroke in Patients With Atrial Fibrillation

	Condition	Points
C	Congestive heart failure	1
H	Hypertension >140/90 mm Hg	1
A_2	Age ≥75	2
D	Diabetes mellitus	1
S_2	Prior stroke or transient ischemic attack	2
V	Prior vascular disease (MI, peripheral vascular disease)	1
A	Age 65–74	1
Sc	Female sex	1

Clinical Presentation: Can be paroxysmal or chronic. Patients can be asymptomatic or have symptoms ranging from palpitations, chest discomfort, lightheadedness, and syncope to hemodynamic instability. Can also occur secondary to MI or stroke:

- Atrial fibrillation with rapid ventricular response indicates rapid conduction through the AV node and ↑ventricular rate
- Long-standing tachycardia can lead to dilated cardiomyopathy

PPx: Preventable risk factors: obesity

MoD: Ectopic atrial conduction originating from around the pulmonary veins

- Causes of atrial fibrillation include but are not limited to: structural heart disease, valvular heart disease (mitral regurgitation, mitral stenosis), asthma and COPD, hyperthyroidism, hypertension, obstructive sleep apnea, and alcohol consumption.

Dx:

1. EKG showing absence of P-waves and irregularly irregular rhythm.
2. Holter monitor for paroxysmal atrial fibrillation.

Tx/Mgmt:

1. Hemodynamically unstable → synchronized cardioversion
2. Hemodynamically stable:
   - Onset less than 48 hours
3. Rate control—β-blockers (metoprolol), non-dihydropyridine CCBs (verapamil, diltiazem):
   - Onset greater than 48 hours
     - Use CHA_2DS_2-VASc
   - Score of 0 in males or 1 in females → no anticoagulation needed
   - Score of 1 in males → consider anticoagulation
   - Score ≥2 → anticoagulate
4. Consider rate control, rhythm control (class I and III antiarrhythmics), synchronized cardioversion, or catheter ablation (of the electrical pathways near the pulmonary veins)

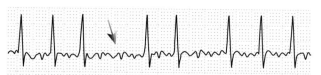

FIG. 7.3 Atrial fibrillation. (From https://en.wikipedia.org/wiki/Atrial_fibrillation#/media/File:Afib_ecg.jpg.)

Infectious and Inflammatory Disorders

Acute Pericarditis

Buzz Words: Friction rub + diffuse ST-elevations with PR-depressions + improvement with sitting up and leaning forward

Clinical Presentation:
- Sharp chest pain that is classically improved while sitting up and leaning forward
- Diffuse ST-elevations and PR-depressions in all leads except aVR on EKG
- Pericardial friction rub on auscultation

MoD: Inflammation of the pericardium 2/2 infection, uremia, autoimmune (Dressler syndrome), or post-MI/pericardiotomy syndrome

Dx:
1. Clinical presentation + EKG changes
2. GC: Note that patients with uremic pericarditis (usually with blood urea nitrogen [BUN] ≥ 60 mg/dL) often do not have classic EKG changes.

Tx/Mgmt:
1. Nonsteroidal anti-inflammatory drugs (NSAIDs) ± colchicine → steroids
2. Treatment of underlying cause in uremia or autoimmune disease

Constrictive Pericarditis

Buzz Words: Pericardial calcification

Clinical Presentation:
- Hypotension, syncope
- Kussmaul sign = ↑ in jugular vein distention (JVD) with inspiration
- Pericardial calcification
- Pericardial knock (early diastolic sound) on auscultation

MoD: Calcification and fibrosis of the pericardium leading to diastolic dysfunction and impaired filling
- Developed countries—viral (coxsackievirus, echovirus adenovirus), radiation, cardiac surgery
- Undeveloped countries—tuberculosis

Dx: Echocardiography showing calcifications and elevated diastolic pressures

Tx/Mgmt: Pericardiotomy

Infectious Endocarditis

Buzz Words: Splinter hemorrhage + Roth spots + Janeway lesions + Osler nodes

Clinical Presentation:
- Fever, malaise
- Splinter hemorrhage, Roth spots (retinal hemorrhage with pale center), Janeway lesions (painless microabscess/embolus), Osler nodes (Osler = Ouch!; painful nodules in fingers—immune complex)
- Embolic disease—stroke, arterial occlusion, seeding of bacteria causing local infection (Fig. 7.4)

MoD:
- Native valve—*Staphylococcus aureus*
- Damaged valves—*Staphylococcus epidermidis*, *S. aureus*
- Dental procedures—**Viridans group streptococci** (*Streptococcus mutans*, *Streptococcus mitis*, *Streptococcus sanguinis*)
- IVDU—*S. aureus*, *Candida*, *Pseudomonas*
- GU procedures—*Enterococci*
- Colon cancer—*Streptococcus gallolyticus* (***Streptococcus bovis***), *Clostridium septicum*
- Culture negative infectious endocarditis—**HACEK** organisms (although some are now able to be cultured), *Coxiella*, *Bartonella*, *Chlamydia*

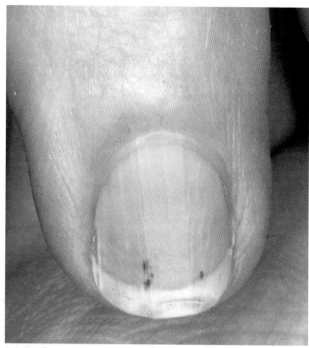

FIG. 7.4 Splinter hemorrhages. (From https://en.wikipedia.org/wiki/Splinter_hemorrhage.)

Dx:
1. Large-volume blood cultures
2. Echocardiography

Tx/Mgmt: Antibiotics ± surgical debridement/valve replacement

Non-Infectious (Marantic endocarditis)

Buzz Words: Sterile vegetations on cardiac valves associated with malignancy and autoimmune disease

Clinical Presentation:
- Sterile deposits on cardiac valves → can flick off and cause thrombotic disease
- Libman-Sacks endocarditis is associated with systemic lupus erythematosus and presents with deposits on both the atrial and ventricular surfaces of cardiac valves:
  - Most commonly causes valve dysfunction → embolic disease

Dx: Echocardiography

Tx/Mgmt:
1. Anticoagulation with warfarin.
2. Treatment of underlying disease.
3. Surgical valve repair/replacement.

Diseases of Vascular System

Orthostatic Hypotension

Buzz Words: Syncope + decrease in systolic blood pressure (BP) of ≥20 mm Hg or diastolic BP of ≥10 mm Hg when moving from supine to sitting to standing position

Clinical Presentation: Dizziness, lightheadedness, syncope, temporary decrease in vision or hearing

PPx: N/A

MoD: Intravascular volume depletion, autonomic dysfunction (diabetes mellitus, multiple system atrophy), medication side effect (tricyclic antidepressants, α1-antagonists [doxazosin, prazosin, tamsulosin, terazosin])

Dx: Orthostatic vital signs: decrease in systolic BP of ≥20 mm Hg or diastolic BP of ≥10 mm Hg taken 3 minutes after moving from supine to sitting to standing position

Tx/Mgmt:
1. Increase fluid intake.
2. Medications to increase blood pressure: midodrine (α1-agonist), dopamine antagonists, tyramine, indomethacin.

Hypertension

Buzz Words: BP ≥140/90 mm Hg

Clinical Presentation: Very high-yield. Insidious and asymptomatic until secondary effects become evident. Patients with hypertension have increased risk for cardiovascular disease, renal disease, and stroke. The most important concept to learn for the family medicine shelf is the screening criteria for hypertension.

PPx: Per USPSTF, screening criteria for hypertension: (1) Annual screening for adults older than 40 years or those at high risk (i.e., 130–139/85–89 BP, overweight, or African-Americans). (2) Adults aged 18–39 years with BP less than 130/85 mm Hg with no other risk factors should have BP checked every 3–5 years.

Link to USPSTF guidelines for hypertension screening

MoD: May be primary (idiopathic/essential) or secondary to other pathology
- Causes of secondary hypertension include:
  - Chronic renal failure
  - Renal artery stenosis—classically in older males with a history of atherosclerotic disease
  - Fibromuscular dysplasia—classically in younger women
  - High yield for family medicine shelf
  - Hyperaldosteronism—via increased sodium absorption in the distal convoluted tubule
  - Hyper- or hypothyroidism—via hyperdynamic circulation (hyperthyroidism) or vasoconstriction (hypothyroidism)
  - Obstructive sleep apnea
  - Others—scleroderma, pheochromocytoma

Dx:
1. Measurement of blood pressure on two separate occasions; hypertension is currently considered the following:
   - Over age 60 → 150/90
   - Under age 60 → 140/90
   - With CKD, any age → 140/90
   - With diabetes, any age → 140/90
2. Diagnosis of renal artery stenosis and fibromuscular dysplasia through CT angiogram

Tx/Mgmt:
1. Lifestyle modification—weight loss, reduce dietary sodium
2. Medication:
   a. In patients with CKD → start with ACE inhibitor or ARB

b. In patients without CKD
   i. If African-American → HCTZ or CCB
   ii. Otherwise → HCTZ or ACE inhibitor or ARB or CCB
c. BP goals (if either SBP or DBP is over indicated value, must treat)
   i. Over age 60 → <150/90
   ii. Under age 60 → <140/90
   iii. With CKD, any age → <140/90
   iv. With diabetes, any age → <140/90
d. Reassess every 6 months, do not use ACEI + ARB together in same patient

Peripheral Artery Disease

Buzz Words: Cool, pale extremities with weak or absent pulses + loss of hair + shiny skin

Clinical Presentation:
- Cool, pale extremities, weak/absent pulses, loss of hair, atrophy, necrosis, gangrene
- Intermittent limb claudication (pain with activity)
- GC: Claudication is to the limb and angina is to the heart

PPx:
- Management of risk factors—abstain from **smoking**, control of DM, HLD, and HTN

MoD:
- Destruction or chronic occlusive disease of peripheral vessels → ↓ perfusion of extremities
- Smoking damages the vascular endothelium and promotes atherosclerotic changes

Dx:
1. Ankle brachial index (ABI) ≤0.9:
   - GC: Patients with calcification of the peripheral vasculature may have falsely elevated ABI
2. Duplex ultrasound and Doppler studies

Tx/Mgmt:
1. Smoking cessation, management of comorbid conditions:
   a. Cessation of smoking prevents further accelerated vascular disease but does not necessarily significantly improve existing vascular pathology
2. Supervised exercise program
3. Medications—cilostazol (antiplatelet + vasodilator), pentoxifylline
4. Surgical intervention—angioplasty, stenting, bypass, thrombolysis

Compartment Syndrome

Buzz Words: Pain + pulselessness + paresthesias + paralysis + pallor + poikilothermia + compartment pressures ≥30 mm Hg

Clinical Presentation:

- 6Ps—pain, pulselessness, paresthesias, paralysis, pallor, poikilothermia (difference in temperature between affected segment and surrounding areas)
- Complications include permanent muscle or nerve damage → rhabdomyolysis

MoD:

- Etiologies include:
    - Bleeding into a limb
    - Crush injuries (tissue edema + bleeding)
    - Ischemic reperfusion injury
    - Tissue swelling after casting

Dx:

1. Diagnosis is typically by clinical presentation.
2. Intra-compartmental pressure ≥30 mm Hg is suggestive.

Tx/Mgmt: Fasciotomy

Deep Vein Thrombosis

Buzz Words: Swelling and pain of a limb with limb asymmetry, Homan sign

Clinical Presentation:

- Swelling, pain, redness of the affected limb ± engorgement of superficial veins
- Homan sign = pain with dorsiflexion of the foot (this test is historical and is not sensitive or specific)

PPx:

- Ambulation, compression stockings, anticoagulation (heparin or enoxaparin)

MoD:

- Most commonly occurs in the proximal deep veins of the lower extremities (femoral veins, popliteal veins, iliac veins)
- Risk factors include: hypercoagulable state (factor V Leiden, malignancy, recent surgery, hormone replacement therapy), endothelial cell damage, and venous stasis

Dx:

1. Duplex ultrasound.
2. D-dimer—can be used to rule out deep vein thrombosis (DVT) if negative.

Tx/Mgmt:
1. Provoked DVT—an underlying factor can be identified to explain the DVT (e.g., concurrent malignancy, prior immobilization, recent surgery):
   a. Anticoagulation with warfarin or low-molecular-weight heparin for 3 months
2. Unprovoked DVT—no underlying factor can be identified:
   a. Anticoagulation with warfarin for 3–6 months for first episode
   b. Anticoagulation for 12 months to indefinite for second episode
3. Inferior vena cava filter (if patient is unable to tolerate anticoagulation)

Venous Insufficiency

Buzz Words: Lower extremity edema with evidence of stasis dermatitis ± prominent varicose veins due to venous valvular insufficiency
Clinical Presentation:
- Lower extremity edema with hyperpigmentation, scaling, and shiny, indurated appearance of the skin (**stasis dermatitis**)
- Prominent varicose veins
- Lipodermatosclerosis = chronic panniculitis (inflammation of fat) with sclerosis and inverted champagne bottle appearance of the lower leg

MoD:
- Dysfunction or destruction of venous valves leads to backflow and pooling in the dependent veins of the body

Dx: Based on history and clinical exam
Tx/Mgmt:
1. Compression stockings
2. Leg elevation
3. Disorders of the great vessels

Aortic Aneurysm (Thoracic and Abdominal)

Buzz Words: Widened mediastinum → thoracic aortic aneurysm
Pulsatile abdominal mass → abdominal aortic aneurysm (AAA)
Clinical Presentation:
- AAA—pulsatile abdominal mass:
  - Risk factors include: atherosclerosis, smoking, and hypertension
- Thoracic aortic aneurysm—widened mediastinum on chest radiograph:
  - Risk factors include: smoking, hypertension, and atherosclerosis

- GC: Patients with connective tissue disease (Marfan syndrome, Ehlers-Danlos syndrome, Loeys-Dietz syndrome) as well as those with syphilitic aortitis are at increased risk for thoracic aortic aneurysms.

MoD: Weakening of the vascular wall (through atherosclerosis or intrinsic defects in collagen and support proteins) leads to ballooning and formation of an aneurysm

Dx:

1. Male smokers between 65- and 75-years old should be screened with a one-time abdominal ultrasound.
2. Echocardiogram or CT angiogram for thoracic aortic aneurysms.
3. CT angiogram can also be used for accurate assessment of AAAs.

Tx/Mgmt:

1. Modification of risk factors—statins, smoking cessation, and control of blood pressure
2. Surgical treatment is indicated for those at higher risk for rupture:
   a. AAA—diameter greater than 5.5 cm, rate of growth greater than 1 cm/year, current smokers
   b. Thoracic aortic aneurysm—aneurysms greater than 5–6 cm

Aortic Dissection

Buzz Words: Tearing chest pain that radiates to the back
Clinical Presentation:

- Acute onset, severe, tearing chest pain that radiates to the back
- May be associated with hypertension or hypotension, aortic insufficiency, acute MI, or acute stroke depending on location and progression of dissection
- Dissection of the subclavian artery may lead to different blood pressure readings between arms

PPx:

- Blood pressure control

MoD:

- Tearing of the tunica intima of the aorta → blood flow between the layers of the aorta leading to dissection
- Risk factors include: **hypertension**, collagen vascular disease (Marfan syndrome, Ehlers-Danlos syndrome), bicuspid aortic valve, and tertiary syphilis

Dx:

1. **Transesophageal echocardiography** is the diagnostic test of choice because of speed
   a. **Magnetic resonance imaging** is the gold standard (more sensitive and equal specificity compared to CT angiography)
   b. Aortography is not typically used anymore
2. **CT angiography** is often used in the emergent setting because of high sensitivity and speed
3. Chest X-ray may show widened mediastinum

Tx/Mgmt:

1. Blood pressure control with β-blockers (labetalol) or CCBs ± nitroprusside.
2. Dissection of the ascending aorta (Stanford type A) → surgery.
3. Dissection of the descending aorta (Stanford type B) → medical management.

QUICK TIPS

Leriche syndrome = atherosclerotic disease of the descending aorta and aortic bifurcation that presents with the triad of: Leg claudication, Impotence, Muscle atrophy

Cholesterol Abnormalities

Hyperlipidemia

Buzz Words: High LDL cholesterol or low HDL cholesterol

Clinical Presentation: Hypercholesterolemia is one of the most important diseases on the family medicine shelf. This is a condition characterized by high levels of cholesterol in the blood. Whereas there are few acute complications of just having these high levels of cholesterol, it can lead to plaque formation in coronary arteries and peripheral arteries, leading to occlusion and ischemia/infarction. High cholesterol levels can often be visualized in the eyes or in tissue around the body as xanthelasma/xanthoma.

Be sure to learn the screening guidelines and remember that the recommendations are different for men and women (women get screened later).

PPx: According to the USPSTF, guidelines for hyperlipidemia include: (1) Screen men older than 35 years. (2) Screen men 20–35 years if and only if they are at increased risk of coronary heart disease. (3) Screen women older than 45 years if at increased risk of coronary heart disease. (4) Screen women 20–45 years of age if at risk of coronary heart disease. (5) No recommendation made for or against screening in men 20–35 years old and women younger than 20 years who do NOT have an increased risk of coronary heart disease. (6) No screening if patient is younger than 20 years.

Can prevent hyperlipidemia through:

1. Diet and exercise
2. Low-fat diets

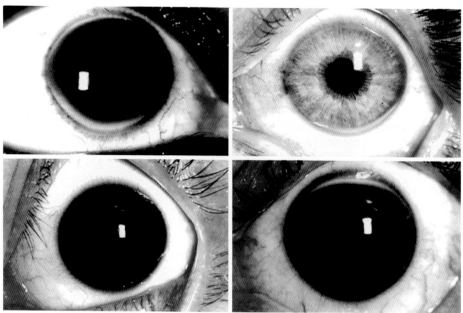

FIG. 7.5 Corneal arcus. Deposition of cholesterol in the limbic area of the pupil resulting in a white ring seen in hypercholesterolemia and in the elderly. (From https://en.wikipedia.org/wiki/Arcus_senilis.)

 AR

Recommendation for use of statins

99 AR

Effectiveness of Statins

MoD: Caused by a combination of diet/genetics

Dx:

1. History and physical (may notice corneal arcus or xanthelasma)
2. Lipid panel (e.g., serum LDL, HDL)

Tx/Mgmt:

1. Lifestyle modification
2. Statin therapy (Figs. 7.5 and 7.6)

HMG CO-A REDUCTASE INHIBITORS-STATINS

Agent	Doses (mg)	LDL↓	HDL↑	Trig↓
Lovastatin	10, 20, 40, (80)	21%–32%	5%–8%	13%–19% (225)
Pravastatin	10, 20, 40, (80)	20%–30%	3%–6%	8%–13% (226)
Simvastatin	5, 10, 20, 40, 80	26%–45%	5%–7%	12%–18% (227)
Fluvastatin	20, 40, 80 (XL)	22%–36%	3%–7%	12%–19% (228)
Atorvastatin	10, 20, 40, 80	39%–60%	5%–12%	19%–37% (229)
Rosuvastatin	5, 10, 20, 40	45%–63%	8%–13%	23%–35% (230)

Familial Hypercholesterolemia

Buzz Words: Early atherosclerotic disease, tendon xanthoma, increased serum cholesterol

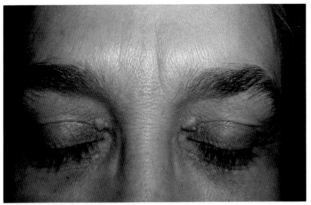

FIG. 7.6 Xanthelasma. Note the yellow-hued papules around the eyelids representing deposits of cholesterol. May be seen in patients with hypercholesterolemia but may also be seen in normo-cholesterolemic patients. (From https://en.wikipedia.org/wiki/Xanthelasma.)

Clinical Presentation: Early atherosclerotic disease (CAD, MI, PAD), tendon xanthoma, corneal arcus, xanthelasma

MoD: Mutation in the LDL receptor or ApoB that results in ability of the liver to clear cholesterol from the blood

Dx:
1. Total serum cholesterol:
   - 350–550 mg/dL is suggestive of heterozygous state
   - 650–1000 mg/dL is suggestive of homozygous state
2. Mutation analysis

Tx/Mgmt:
1. Homozygous mutants—high dose statins + lipid apheresis, liver transplant.
2. Heterozygous mutants—statins ± bile acid sequestrants (cholestyramine), niacin.

Familial Hyperchylomicronemia (Lipoprotein Lipase Deficiency)

Buzz Words: Creamy layer in supernatant of blood sample + serum fasting triglycerides

Clinical Presentation: Eruptive xathomas, acute pancreatitis (due to ⇈ triglycerides)
   - No increased risk of atherosclerotic disease

MoD: Caused by deficiency in lipoprotein lipase

Dx:
1. Blood testing showing increased fasting triglycerides greater than 1000 mg/dL
2. Milky, creamy plasma with increased hyperchylomicronemia.

Tx/Mgmt:
1. Low-fat diet and avoidance of simple carbohydrates.
2. Lipid lowering medications—omega-3-fatty acids, gemfibrozil

Familial Hypertriglyceridemia

Buzz Words: Triglycerides greater than 1000 mg/dL
Clinical Presentation: Presents with xanthoma, corneal arcus, xanthelasma, and acute pancreatitis (due to ↑↑ triglycerides); increased risk of pancreatitis (triglycerides >1000 mg/dL)
MoD: Mutations in the ApoA5 and lipase I genes
Dx: Fasting serum triglycerides greater than 1000 mg/dL
Tx/Mgmt:
1. Low-fat diet and avoidance of simple carbohydrates.
2. Lipid-lowering medications—omega-3 fatty acids, gemfibrozil.

GUNNER PRACTICE

1. A 36-year-old man with type II diabetes presents to your clinic for an annual wellness visit. His physical exam is unremarkable, but his BMI is 42.5. His father died of cardiovascular disease at the age of 50 and his mother and grandmother both had breast cancer. He does not drink alcohol or smoke cigarettes. You notice that his blood pressure has been 145/95 on a visit 3 months ago and today it is 150/95. Which of the following is the most appropriate next step in management?
   A. No management needed
   B. Dietary counseling
   C. Pharmacologic intervention for hypertension
   D. CAGE questionnaire
   E. ECG

2. A 54-year-old man presents to your office with sharp chest pain 1 month after he was hospitalized for a myocardial infarction. He notes the pain has gotten worse over the past week and gets worse when he leans forward. Cardiac auscultation is normal, although you notice ST elevation in all leads on his EKG. Which of the following is the most appropriate next step in management?
   A. Emergency room referral
   B. NSAID prescription
   C. Electrocardiogram
   D. Psychiatric evaluation
   E. No management necessary

Notes

ANSWERS: What Would Gunner Jess/Jim Do?

1. WWGJD? A 36-year-old man with type II diabetes presents to your clinic for an annual wellness visit. His physical exam is unremarkable, but his BMI is 42.5. His father died of cardiovascular disease at the age of 50 and his mother and grandmother both had breast cancer. He does not drink alcohol or smoke cigarettes. You notice that his blood pressure has been 145/95 on a visit 3 months ago and today it is 150/95. Which of the following is the most appropriate next step in management?

Answer: C. Pharmacologic intervention for hypertension.

   Explanation: Patients with CKD or chronic kidney disease at any age should be treated when blood pressure is above 140/90. A consistently raised blood pressure both of which are above these limits suggests pharmacologic treatment is necessary. This patient should be started with an ACE inhibitor, which is indicated for the treatment of both hypertension and diabetes.

   A. No management needed → Incorrect. There is a clear need for management both for hypertension and morbid obesity (obesity III) in this patient.

   B. Dietary counseling → Incorrect. Whereas this is also indicated as the patient has a high BMI, the more pressing issue is the treatment of hypertension, which exceeds limits and warrants pharmacologic intervention.

   D. CAGE questionnaire → Incorrect. There is no evidence this patient is attempting to deceive when he says he does not drink alcohol and thus CAGE questionnaire is not indicated.

   E. ECG → Incorrect. There is no evidence of any cardiac pathology and thus an electroencephalogram is not needed. This would be indicated for an arrhythmia or MI.

2. WWGJD? A 54-year-old man presents to your office with sharp chest pain 1 month after he was hospitalized for a myocardial infarction. He notes the pain has gotten worse over the past week and gets worse when he leans forward. Cardiac auscultation is normal, although you notice ST elevation in all leads on his EKG. Which of the following is the most appropriate next step in management?

Answer: B. NSAID prescription.

   Explanation: Pericarditis can occur after myocardial infarction. A classical presenting sign is sharp chest pain that gets worse when leaning forward. You may not always hear a friction rub on auscultation, although persistent ST elevation is a giveaway toward pericarditis—note you differentiate pericarditis from MI based on ST elevation in all leads or a specific set of leads. NSAIDs are the first line of treatment for pericarditis.

A. Emergency room referral → This patient is unlikely to be having a repeat myocardial infarction because his pain has gotten worse over the past week and gets worse when he leans forward. ST elevation in all leads is not consistent with STEMI.

C. Electrocardiogram → This patient is unlikely to be having a repeat myocardial infarction because his pain has gotten worse over the past week and gets worse when he leans forward. ST elevation in all leads is not consistent with STEMI. ECG would be indicated if this were an MI.

D. Psychiatric evaluation → This would be indicated if this patient were suspected to be malingering or have factitious disorder. There is no evidence that this is happening.

E. No management necessary → This person is in clear pain and warrants management.

Diseases of the Respiratory System

Leo Wang, William Plum, Lauren Briskie, Hao-Hua Wu, and Katherine Margo

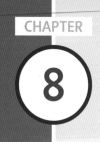

Introduction

Diseases of the respiratory system are more than fair game for the Family Medicine Shelf and comprise 5%–10% of your exam. The respiratory system includes upper and lower airways, lungs, pleura, and the diaphragm. We will introduce and cover various pathologies in these categories. However, not all topics are covered equally. Some of the higher yield topics, upon which we will focus with a heavier hand in this chapter, are worth giving your time to achieve mastery. The most high-yield topic that will be tested on the Family Medicine Shelf is asthma. Focus on every aspect of asthma from prophylactic (PPx) to treatment/management (Tx/Mgmt). The second most high-yield topic in this chapter is upper respiratory infections (URIs).

Disorders of the Lung Parenchyma

Alpha-1 Antitrypsin Deficiency

Buzz Words: Emphysema/bronchiectasis + young adult + occasional smoker or non-smoker + neonatal cholestatic jaundice + cirrhosis + liver cancer + panniculitis

Clinical Presentation: Alpha-1 antitrypsin inhibits neutrophil elastase in order to protect the lung from protease-mediated destruction. When alpha-1 antitrypsin is deficient or its activity cannot keep up with the amount of damage done, neutrophile elastase activity is upregulated, leading to destruction of lung tissue (e.g., early emphysema). In addition, alpha-1 antitrypsin is also contained in the liver, causing pathology if there is a defect in the enzyme. Defective alpha-1 antitrypsin, for instance, could be stuck in the hepatocytes that they are made in leading to jaundice, cirrhosis, and eventually liver cancer due to increased risk. Thus, suspect this disease in patients who develop emphysema/liver pathology when they are young.

PPx: (1) Smoking cessation (avoiding any insult to lungs)

Mechanism of Disease (MoD): (1) Alpha-1 antitrypsin can be deficient due to a decreased in production or abnormal protein

Diagnostic Steps (Dx):
1. Chest X-ray (CXR)
2. Serum alpha-1 antitrypsin levels
3. Genotyping (confirmation of diagnosis)

Tx/Mgmt:
1. Smoking cessation
2. Alpha-1 antitrypsin replacement
3. Liver transplant

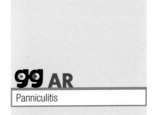

Panniculitis

Cystic Fibrosis

Buzz Words: Bronchiectasis + pneumonia with staph/ pseudo + hypoxia = barrel chest + clubbing + chronic rhinosinusitis + bilateral nasal polyps leading to nasal obstruction/chronic rhinosinusitis + foul-smelling stool (failure to absorb vitamin ADEK) + failure to thrive (2/2 to know fat absorption) → cystic fibrosis (CF):
- Clubbing = bulbous enlargement of the tips of the digits
- Nasal polyps in 40% of CF

CF + Infertility (95% of males, 20% females) + osteopenia/kyphoscoliosis/digital clubbing + meconium ileus/ distal obstruction syndrome + exocrine pancreatic insufficiency + diabetes + recurrent pulmonary pathology → complications of CF

Clinical Presentation: CF is a congenital multiorgan disorder that primarily affects the lung and the pancreas. The chloride channels in CF are defective, meaning that fluid is not sent toward the respiratory or gastrointestinal lumen, and secretions that were meant to be cleared are stuck, leading to infection and digestive abnormality. CF is one of the most high yield diseases on the shelf because it can present in so many different ways in many different age groups. Most notably, patients with CF frequently get pneumonia infected by organisms associated with immunocompromised patients, such as *Pneumocystis jiroveci*. Also, CF patients may have difficulty with digestion owing to a lack of exocrine secretions from the pancreas. Importantly, the treatment for patients with CF is multifaceted and requires a lot of work on the part of the patient. Chest PT, for instance, requires the patient's care provider to tap methodically on the patient's chest to loosen up secretions every single day. Lastly, for the purposes of the shelf, remember that CF is associated with infertility due to no semen production (male) or obstruction of semen entrance (female).

PPx: (1) Screening done as part of newborn screening test in the United States

MoD: Mutation of the CFTR protein → defective chloride ion channels → increased loss of sodium in sweat

For mechanism of infertility → congenital bilateral absence of vas deferens in males, inspissated mucus in the fetal genital tract obstructs developing vas deferens:

- Even if the testes are descended and spermatogenesis is normal → sperm cannot be ejaculated resulting in no semen production (obstructive azoospermia); in females, viscous cervical mucus can obstruct sperm entry.

Dx:

1. CXR
2. Spirometry
3. Quantitative pilocarpine iontophoresis for measurement of sweat chloride concentration; Pilocarpine = cholinergic drug that induces sweating; a chloride level greater than 60 mmol/L on two occasions confirms diagnosis, DNA test to identify two CF mutations
4. F/u with DNA analysis
5. Nasal potential difference (defective nasal epithelial ion transport) → perform if sweat testing and DNA analysis equivocal
6. Sputum culture if pneumonia

Tx/Mgmt:

1. Supportive (steroids for rhinosinusitis or surgery for nasal polyps)
2. Antibiotics for infections (i.e., gentamicin)
3. Lung physiotherapy

Infectious, Immunologic, and Inflammatory Disorders of the Upper Airway

URIs are illnesses caused by infections of the upper respiratory tract, which include the nose, sinuses, pharynx, and larynx. Some terms to be familiar with are the following:

Rhinitis: inflammation of the nasal mucosa

Rhinosinusitis: inflammation of nasal mucosa + sinus mucosa

Nasopharyngitis: inflammation of nasal mucosa + pharynx/uvula/tonsils, aka the common cold

Pharyngitis: inflammation of pharynx/uvula/tonsils

Epiglottitis: inflammation of the epiglottis
Laryngitis: inflammation of the larynx
Laryngotracheitis: inflammation of larynx, trachea
Tracheitis: inflammation of trachea and subglottic area
    A number of bacterial and viral etiologies exist for each of these different pathologies and are discussed below.

Acute Nasopharyngitis

Buzz Words: Daycare/childcare + sniffling + runny nose/congestion + sneezing + sore throat + winter + cough + no/low fever

Clinical Presentation: Whereas viral etiologies of the common cold will traditionally cause nasopharyngitis, it can manifest with any of the pathologies above, including pharyngitis, rhinitis, or even sinusitis. The average adult gets up to 4–5 colds a year, whereas children may get as many as 10.

PPx: Adequate hand hygiene, reduce stress, stay away from the sick, and do not touch eyes/mouth/nose with bare hands; some controversy exists over Zn or vitamin C supplementation. Vaccination is ineffective.

MoD: Most common viral etiology is rhinovirus, which spread through air via close contacts with infected people and for indirect contact with objects in environment → nose/mouth/eyes via droplets. Other causes of the common cold include adenovirus, coronavirus, coxsackievirus, parainfluenza, and RSV. RSV is very common in babies and can cause more severe symptoms. Parainfluenza is second most common in babies and children. Both RSV/parainfluenza can lead to hospitalization.

Dx: Clinical

Tx/Mgmt:
1. Nonsteroidal anti-inflammatory drugs (NSAIDs)/Tylenol
2. Antibiotics should **not** be prescribed
3. Ribavirin/corticosteroids in severe cases

QUICK TIPS

Colds that do not resolve in 2 weeks or get better and then worsen should suspect **bacterial superinfection.**

QUICK TIPS

Coxsackievirus will also cause hand-foot-mouth disease (blisters and rash)

Influenza ("The Flu")

Buzz Words: Lack of vaccinations + sniffling + runny nose/congestion + sneezing + sore throat + winter + muscle ache + fatigue + high fever + chest tightness

Clinical Presentation: The flu is caused by the influenza virus. Differentiate a cold from influenza by the presence of a high fever and **myalgias.** In children, the flu can also cause nausea and vomiting. Some prominent

Symptoms of
Influenza

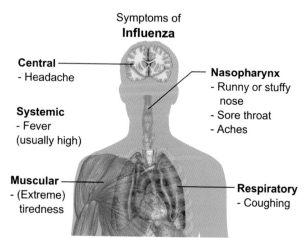

Central
- Headache

Systemic
- Fever
(usually high)

Muscular
- (Extreme)
  tiredness

Nasopharynx
- Runny or stuffy
  nose
- Sore throat
- Aches

Respiratory
- Coughing

FIG. 8.1 Symptoms of influenza (Wiki).

complications include viral pneumonia, bacterial pneumonia, or superinfections leading to bacterial sinusitis. The flu causes 500,000 deaths a year (Fig. 8.1).

PPx: (1) Frequent hand washing, (2) annual influenza vaccine (according to the Centers for Disease Control and Prevention [CDC], everyone 6 months or older should get the vaccine by October)

MoD: Respiratory droplet transmission of influenza A, B, or C. Influenza A is most common and includes the H1N1 to H7N9 viruses. Viruses bind to hemagglutinin on epithelial cells → replication. Neuraminidase leads to release of viral particles from host cells.

Dx:
1. Clinical
2. Rapid influenza test only in severe cases:
   - Variable sensitivity (10%–70%)
3. Other tests exist (polymerase chain reaction [PCR], antigen detection, viral culture) but only used when absolutely critical to make influenza diagnosis (like in healthcare worker, etc.)

Tx/Mgmt:
1. Tylenol/NSAIDS (avoid NSAIDs in children)
2. Neuraminidase inhibitors (oseltamivir, zanamivir)
   - Jury is still out on whether these are helpful in patients without other risk factors
   - AAFP states administration of antivirals based on clinical suspicion before waiting for test results and within 48 hours of symptoms
3. M2 inhibitors (amantadine, rimantadine)
   - Used very infrequently

Sinusitis

Buzz Words: Cold-like symptoms + runny/stuffy noise + facial pain + tenderness over sinuses + nasal polyps:

Tooth pain → maxillary sinusitis

Forehead pain → frontal sinusitis

Eye pain → sphenoidal sinusitis

Pain between eyes/upper nose → ethmoidal sinusitis

Clinical Presentation: Sinusitis occurs mostly due to infection but can also be caused by allergies, smoking, and in children can be caused by pacifier use or bottle drinking while supine. Untreated sinusitis can lead to meningitis or abscess formation.

Three subtypes:

Acute: <4 weeks

Subacute: 4–12 weeks

Chronic: >12 weeks

PPx: Smoking cessation and frequent handwashing

MoD: Viral or bacterial infection of sinuses, leading to swelling/congestion and blocked drainage ducts. Most common acute are viral causes, including rhinovirus, coronavirus, parainfluenza, RSV, enteroviruses, and metapneumovirus. Common bacterial causes include *Streptococcus pneumoniae*, *Haemophilus influenzae*, and *Moraxella catarrhalis*.

Dx:

1. Physical exam
2. Nasal cultures in chronic sinusitis
3. Endoscopy

Tx/Mgmt:

1. OTC decongestant
2. Saline flushes (Neti pot, etc.)
3. Antibiotic course:
   - Amoxicillin first-line, switch to Amox + Clavulanate if does not improve after 7 days
   - Clarithromycin/doxy for those with penicillin allergies
   - Typical Abx course = 7 days
4. Antihistamines if allergies concomitant
5. If chronic and multiplied failed Abx courses, consider sinus surgery: turbinectomy or balloon sinuplasty

QUICK TIPS

In diabetic with sinusitis, suspect mucormycosis

Epiglottitis

Buzz Words: Child + no HiB vaccination (or foreign immigrant) + difficulty swallowing, hoarse voice + stridor

Clinical Presentation: Typically occurs in children with fever + difficulty swallowing. Is caused by HiB or other bacterial infections of the epiglottis. Stridor is upper airway obstruction and is a surgical emergency. Since advent of HiB vaccination, now mostly occurs in older children and adults.

PPx: (1) Vaccinate against HiB, (2) can also use rifampin for people who may have been exposed

MoD: Traditionally caused by HiB, but if immunized, suspect *S. pneumoniae, Streptococcus pyogenes, Staphylococcus aureus.* Also linked to cocaine usage.

Dx:

1. Laryngoscopy to rule out croup, peritonsillar abscess, retropharyngeal abscess
2. X-ray shows thumbprint sign
3. Computed tomography (CT) shows Halloween sign (Fig. 8.2)

Tx/Mgmt:

1. Endotracheal intubation
2. Ceftriaxone + vancomycin
3. Corticosteroids

Croup (Laryngotracheobronchitis)

Buzz Words: Barking cough + coryza + stridor + "steeple sign" on X-ray

Clinical Presentation: Most common in children 6 months to 3 years old and peaks in fall and early winter. Onset is gradual and often begins with rhinorrhea, congestion, and coryza. Proceeds to fever, barking cough, coryza, and inspiratory stridor within next 12–48 hours. Patient will have increased difficulty breathing when lying down.

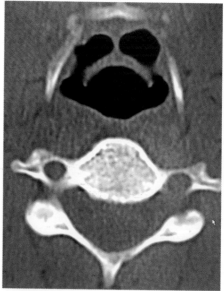

FIG. 8.2 Halloween sign on computed tomography (Wikipedia).

PPx: None

MoD: Most commonly caused by parainfluenza virus types 1 and 2. RSV second most common cause.

Dx: Clinical, may be assisted by finding of narrowed airway on anteroposterior neck radiograph

Tx/Mgmt:

1. Racemic epinephrine for moderate-to-severe cases
2. Supportive treatment and steroids in milder cases

Acute Laryngitis

Buzz Words: Hoarseness with URI symptoms

Clinical Presentation: Commonly seen in children from 5 years through adolescence. Presents with hoarseness, sore throat, rhinorrhea, cough.

PPx: None

MoD: Acute infection causing inflammation of the mucosa of the larynx. Most commonly due to viral respiratory tract infections.

Dx: Clinical

Tx/Mgmt: Usually self-limited process. Treatment is supportive.

Streptococcal Pharyngitis

Buzz Words: Pharyngeal exudates + cervical adenopathy + fever in child

Clinical Presentation: The term tonsillitis may be used in cases when the involvement of the tonsils is prominent. Presents with pain on swallowing, pharyngeal exudates, cervical adenopathy, petechiae, fever greater than 104 °F. Uncommon to have cough or hoarseness. Uncommon in children under 3 years of age.

PPx: None

MoD: Inflammation of the pharynx and adjacent structures. Most commonly caused by group A beta hemolytic strep.

Dx: Rapid strep test. Throat culture is the gold standard for diagnosis

Tx/Mgmt: Oral penicillin or amoxicillin × 10 days. Treatment is necessary to prevent acute rheumatic fever.

Peritonsillar Abscess

Buzz Words: Muffled voice + severe sore throat + drooling + trismus + deviation of the uvula

Clinical Presentation: Most frequently seen in adolescents and young adults. Presents with severe sore throat, drooling, trismus, hot potato/muffled voice. Commonly presents with high fever.

PPx: Prompt treatment of strep infections

MoD: Collection of pus located between the palatine tonsil and the pharyngeal muscles. Often polymicrobial, predominantly caused by group A streptococcal infection, *Staphylococcus*, and respiratory anaerobes.

Dx: Clinical: may see deviation of the uvula to the opposite side of abscess.

Tx/Mgmt:
1. Referral to emergency department
2. Drainage of abscess and antimicrobial therapy

Allergic Rhinitis

Buzz Words: Nasal itching, watery eyes, sneezing + runny nose + congestion

Clinical Presentation: Concomitant with allergies and asthma. Presents with nasal itching, itchy/watery eyes, watery rhinorrhea, nasal congestion, and sneezing. On exam nasal turbinates are pale and edematous. May see allergic shiners—blue/gray discoloration under the eyes and a transverse nasal crease (allergic salute). Symptoms are usually intermittent in response to specific exposures such as cats, pollen.

PPx: Avoidance of allergens

MoD: Histamine release by mast cell degranulation in response to allergens

Dx: IgE testing

Tx/Mgmt: Symptomatic treatment with antihistamines, intranasal steroids

Infectious, Immunologic, and Inflammatory Disorders of the Lower Airway

Pneumonia

Buzz Words: Pleuritic chest pain + onset of fever/chills + crackles/rhonchi/wheezing + dyspnea

Clinical Presentation: Two types of pneumonia:

Community-acquired pneumonia (CAP):
- Most common is *S. pneumonia*
- Occurs in community or within 72 hours of hospitalization
- Typical or atypical
  - Typical
    - *S. pneumoniae* > *H. influenzae* > aerobic GNRs (*Klebsiella*) > *S. aureus*
    - Pleuritic chest pain, thick, purulent sputum
    - Lobar consolidation on X-ray
  - Atypical
    - *Mycoplasma* > *Chlamydia, Coxiella, Legionella*
    - Influenza, adenovirus, parainfluenza, RSV

- No SPUTUM PRODUCTION
- Normal pulse + high fever (pulse-temperature dissociation)
- No consolodation on X-ray, reticulonodular infiltrates everywhere

Nosocomial:
- Hospitalization after 72 hours
- Most common is *Escherichia coli*, pseudomonas, and *S. aureus*

Bronchopneumonia:
- Inflammation of the bronchioles

PPx: Influenza vaccine and pneumococcus vaccine (>65 year olds, patients at high risk, i.e., aseptic)

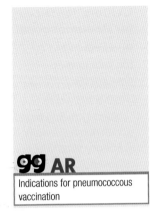

Indications for pneumococcous vaccination

Centers for Disease Control and Prevention Recommendations for Pneumococcal Vaccination

Recommended Groups for Vaccination	Strength	Revaccination
Patients 65 and older	A	Second dose of vaccine if patient received vaccine 5 years or more earlier and was younger than 65 at the time of vaccination
Patients age 2–64 with chronic cardiovascular disease, chronic pulmonary disease, tobacco use, or diabetes mellitus (and patients age 19–64 with asthma)	A	Not recommended
Patients age 2–64 with alcoholism, chronic liver disease, or cerebrospinal fluid leaks	B	Not recommended
Patients age 2–64 with functional or anatomic asplenia	A	If patient is younger than 10, single revaccination 5 years or more after first dose. If patient is 10 or older, consider revaccination 3 years after previous dose.
Patients age 2–64 who live in special environments or social settings including Alaskan natives, American Indians, group homes, nursing homes, prisons, or institutional settings	C	Not recommended

Continued

Centers for Disease Control and Prevention Recommendations for Pneumococcal Vaccination—cont'd

Recommended Groups for Vaccination	Strength	Revaccination
Immunocompromised patients 2 years or older, including those with human immunodeficiency virus infection, leukemia, lymphoma, Hodgkin disease, multiple myeloma, generalized malignancy, chronic renal failure, or nephrotic syndrome; those receiving immunosuppressive chemotherapy (including corticosteroids); and those who have received a transplant	C	Single revaccination if 5 years or more have elapsed since the first dose. If patient is 10 years or younger, consider revaccination 3 years after previous dose.

The following categories reflect the strength of evidence supporting the recommendations for vaccinations; **A** = Strong epidemiologic evidence and substantial clinical benefit support the recommendation for vaccine use. **B** = Moderate evidence supports the recommendation for vaccine use. **C** = Effectiveness of vaccination is not proven, but the high risk for disease and the potential benefits and safely of the vaccine justify vaccination. Strength of evidence for all revaccination recommendations is "C."

MoD: For bacterial pneumonia, the bacteria enter the airway through aspiration of organisms of the nose throat and upper esophagus. Some can also enter the airway through droplets (e.g., Tb and *Legionella*). Bacteria then invade lung parenchyma, leading to inflammatory reaction that is seen clinically and on CXR.

Dx:
1. CBC
2. Blood cultures
3. PA/lateral X-ray
4. Expectorated sputum culture and stain
5. Acid fast for tuberculosis, silver stain for PCP
6. Urinary antigen test for *Legionella*

Tx/Mgmt:
1. Antimicrobial therapy less than 60 (Azithromycin, doxycycline)—outpatient
2. Antimicrobial greater than 60 (levofloxacin, moxifloxacin)—outpatient

3. Hospitalized patients: ceftriaxone + azithromycin
4. Hospital-acquired pneumonia Tx with ceftazidime or imipenem or piperacillin/tazobactam

Fungal Infections

Histoplasmosis

Buzz Words: Ohio and Mississippi River valleys + exposure to bird and bat droppings + erythema nodosum

Clinical Presentation: Most prevalent endemic mycosis in the United States. Found in Ohio and Mississippi River valleys. Most infections are asymptomatic; some individuals develop acute pulmonary infections. Presents with fever, chills, anorexia, cough, and chest pain usually 2–4 weeks after exposure. An extensive exposure can lead to diffuse disease, which can progress to respiratory failure. Often accompanied by joint pain and erythema nodosum.

PPx: None

MoD: *Histoplasma capsulatum* proliferates best in soil contaminated with bird or bat droppings. Organism is inhaled and causes localized or patchy bronchopneumonia. Macrophages are unable to ingest and kill the fungi. Infected macrophages can spread the disease throughout the body.

Dx: Often confused with CAP on CXR. CXR will show focal infiltrates with lymphadenopathy.
1. Clinical
2. CXR/CCT
3. Lesion biopsy
4. Serological
5. PCR
6. Blood culture.

Tx/Mgmt:
1. Most patients recover without treatment
2. In extensive exposure, can treat with anti-fungal therapy: Itraconazole/amphotericin B.

Coccidioidomycosis

Buzz Words: Pneumonia + meningitis

Clinical Presentation: Found in Southwestern United States, northern Mexico, South/Central America. Disease ranges from self-limited acute pneumonia (valley fever) to disseminated disease. More significant illness is correlated to more intensive exposure. Primary infection most frequently manifests as CAP about 21 days after exposure. Most common symptoms are chest pain, cough, and fever. May also present with fatigue, arthralgias, and erythema nodosum.

PPx: None

MoD: Inhalation of spores, usually from stirred up dust

Dx:
1. Clinical
2. CXR/CCT
3. Lesion biopsy
4. Serological
5. PCR
6. Blood culture

Tx/Mgmt:
1. Most patients recover without therapy.
2. Consider antifungal therapy in immunosuppressed patients or those with severe manifestations of disease: Fluconazole, Amphotericin B, Itraconazole.

Blastomycosis

Buzz Words: Pneumonia + skin/bone disease

Clinical Presentation: Shadows histoplasmosis in Midwestern and SE United States

PPx: None

MoD: Inhalation of spores

Dx:
1. Clinical
2. CXR/CCT
3. Lesion biopsy
4. Serological
5. PCR
6. Blood culture

Tx/Mgmt:
1. Itraconazole
2. Amphotericin
3. Fluconazole (Fig. 8.3)

Asthma

Buzz Words: Reversible + cough + wheezing + prolonged expiratory phase + chest pain/tightness + tachypnea + dyspnea

Clinical Presentation: Most common chronic disease of childhood. Exacerbated by viral infections, exposure to allergens and irritants, exercise, changes in weather. Nighttime symptoms are common. Symptoms reversible with bronchodilator therapy differentiates from chronic obstructive pulmonary disease (COPD). Acute exacerbation presents with wheezing, prolonged expiratory phase, chest tightness, tachypnea, and

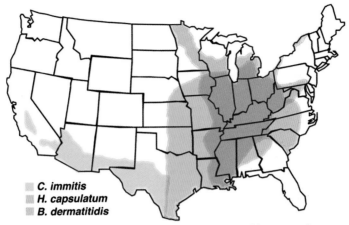

FIG. 8.3 Geographic distribution for *Coccidioides*, *Histoplasma*, and *Blastomycosis*.

dyspnea. Associated with eczema and seasonal allergies (allergic triad).

Classifications of asthma:

Intermittent: symptoms ≤2 days/week

Nighttime awakenings ≤2×/month

Short-acting beta agonist (SABA) use ≤2 days/week

No interference with normal activity

Normal FEV1 between exacerbations, FEV1 >80% predicted, FEV1/FVC normal

Step 1 treatment: Albuterol (SABA) as needed

Mild persistent: symptoms ≥2 days/week, but not daily

Nighttime awakenings 3–4×/month

SABA use >2 days/week, but not daily. Not more than once per day

Minor limitation with activity

Step 2 treatment: SABA + low-dose inhaled glucocorticoid

Moderate persistent: symptoms daily

Nighttime awakenings >1x/week, but not nightly

SABA use daily

Some limitation with activity

Step 3: SABA + medium-dose inhaled corticosteroid

Severe: symptoms throughout the day

Nighttime awakenings: nightly

SABA use several times per day

Extreme limitation of activity

Step 4: SABA + medium-dose inhaled glucocorticoid + long-acting beta agonist (LABA)

Step 5: SABA + high-dose inhaled glucocorticoid + LABA or montelukast (leukotriene antagonist)

In severe cases, can move up to step 6 and add oral systemic glucocorticoids.

PPx: Avoid exposure to triggers, careful adherence to medications

MoD: Inflammatory cells, chemical mediators, and chemotactic factors mediate underlying inflammatory response. Inflammation contributes to airway hyperresponsiveness. Results in edema, increased mucous production, and influx of inflammatory cells. Chronic inflammation leads to airway remodeling.

Dx:

1. Clinical diagnosis based on symptoms!
2. PFTs can assist with diagnosis, but may be normal between exacerbations and are difficult to obtain in young children:

   PFTs: decreased FEV1/FVC, increase in FEV1 greater than 12% with use of albuterol, decrease in FEV1 greater than 20% with methacholine challenge, increased diffusion capacity for the lung for carbon monoxide (DLCO).

   In acute exacerbation: Peak expiratory flow can be used; it is an approximation of FVC.
3. CXR can be obtained to exclude pneumonia, CHF.

Management of asthma: To determine treatment, must first determine classification of asthma. Use stepwise method of treatment as described in "Clinical Presentation." Patient can be moved up or down based on the severity and control of symptoms.

Treatment of acute exacerbation:

1. Best initial therapy = Albuterol via inhaler or nebulizer, systemic steroids, oxygen if hypoxemia:
   a. Ipratropium can be given and is often given in combination with albuterol and has been shown to decrease hospitalization rate for pediatric patients presenting to ED with asthma exacerbation. Ipratropium does not work as quickly as albuterol.
   b. Magnesium can be used to help relieve bronchospasm and can be used in refractory status asthmaticus.
   c. If patient is not responding to treatment and has an increasing PCO$_2$ on ABG, need to consider non-invasive ventilation or intubation.

Chronic Obstructive Pulmonary Disease

Buzz Words: Cough + sputum production + dyspnea

Clinical Presentation: Either chronic bronchitis or emphysema:

Chronic bronchitis:
- Clinical diagnosis, cough + sputum 3 months per year for 2+ years
- Blue bloaters
  - Overweight and cyanotic, chronic cough, cor pulmonale (right heart failure) with no use of accessory muscles and not in respiratory distress

Emphysema:
- Pathologic diagnosis with enlargement of air spaces
- Pink puffers
- Thin, increased energy expenditure during breathing and tend to lean forward with a barrel chest, in obvious distress and uses accessory muscles

Both can coexist

PPx: (1) Smoking cessation or prevent exposure to second-hand smoke, (2) chronic asthma can cause COPD as well, (3) all must get pneumococcus vaccination

MoD: Chronic bronchitis—mucous production narrows airways → inflammation/scarring → obstruction
  Emphysema—increased protease activity from tobacco smoking → breakdown of alveolar walls

Dx:
1. PFT (obstruction FEV1 <70% of normal value, TLC, RV, FRC increased)
2. CXR
   - Low sensitivity, hyperinflammation, flattened diaphragm, diminished vasculature markings
3. ABG

Tx/Mgmt:
1. B2 agonists (albuterol or salmeterol)
2. Inhaled anticholinergics (ipratropium bromide)
3. Corticosteroids (budesonide, fluticasone)
4. Acute exacerbation (persistent increase in sputum and cough → respiratory failure)
   - Bronchodilators + systemic corticosteroids + antibiotics + supplemental O_2
   - Intubation if needed (Fig. 8.4)

Neoplasms

Solitary Pulmonary Nodule

Buzz Words: Singular nodule/lesion, accidental finding

Clinical Presentation: Single, well-defined, round opacity surrounded completely by pulmonary parenchyma, and ≤3 cm. If imaging also depicts atelectasis, lymph node enlargement, or pleural effusion the lesion is not a solitary pulmonary nodule (SPN). Usually found accidently

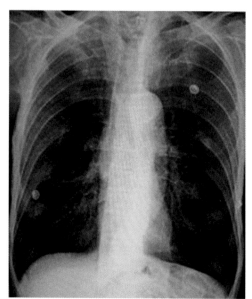

FIG. 8.4 Chronic obstructive pulmonary disease (Wikipedia).

on chest X-ray. For SPN, it is more important to focus on the Dx and Mgmt rather than the cause of the nodule.

PPx: N/A

MoD: (1) Benign neoplasia: hamartoma, fibroma, chondroma, or neural tumor; (2) infectious: tuberculosis, fungal infection, abscess, nocardia, nontuberculosis mycobacteria, round pneumonia, septic embolus; (3) malignant neoplasia: bronchogenic carcinoma, carcinoid/neuroendocrine, metastasis, lymphoma, teratoma, leiomyoma; (4) inflammatory: granulomatosis with polyangiitis, rheumatoid nodule, sarcoidosis; (5) vascular: arteriovenous malformation, hematoma, pulmonary artery aneurysm, pulmonary venous varix, pulmonary infarct; (6) bronchial: bronchogenic cyst, mucocele, lung sequestration

Dx:

1. Compare with previous imaging
2. If low risk for malignancy, or 2-year radiographic stability, no further testing required, and follow yearly with serial chest CT scans
3. If intermediate risk of malignancy, either fine-needle aspiration (FNA) or positron emission tomography (PET) scan is acceptable. If the results suggest malignancy, surgical resection is the next step. However, if the results are nondiagnostic, active surveillance is the correct course of action
4. If high risk for malignancy, surgical excision of nodule is recommended.

QUICK TIPS

Do not forget looking at previous imaging!

Tx/Mgmt:
1. Serial chest CT scans
2. CT-FNA
3. PET scan
4. Surgical excision

Management of SPN

Lip-Squamous Cell Carcinoma

Buzz Words: Smoker + alcohol use + "persistent" papules, plaques, erosions, or ulcers

Clinical Presentation: Exophytic or ulcerative lesion likely associated with pain. Slow-growing, local tumor with a low potential to metastasize.

PPx: (1) Smoking cessation, (2) alcohol cessation, (3) adequate sun protection

MoD: Malignant proliferation of squamous keratinocytes

Dx:
1. Physical exam
2. Biopsy

Tx/Mgmt:
1. Refer to dermatologist
2. Mohs surgery or excision
3. Second-line treatments include topical imiquimod and 5-fluorouracil

QUICK TIPS
Lip SCC is more commonly found on lower lip due to greater sun exposure.

Lung-Squamous Cell Carcinoma

Buzz Words: Smoker + persistent cough + hemoptysis + hypercalcemia + superior vena cava (SVC) syndrome + Horner's

Clinical Presentation: Intrathoracic symptoms of squamous cell carcinoma (SCC) include a persistent cough, hemoptysis, chest pain, dyspnea, hoarseness, and wheezing. Constitutional symptoms, especially in a smoker, such as weight loss, decreased appetite, and weakness should raise your suspicion for lung cancer. Be on the lookout for recurrent pneumonia in the same lobe, as this could be a sign of postobstructive pneumonia.

PPx: (1) Smoking cessation, avoiding asbestos, and avoiding radon; (2) low-dose CT screening for those age 55–77 who have no symptoms and have a 30-pack per year smoking history (controversial)

MoD:
- SCC-malignant proliferation of squamous keratinocytes
- SVC syndrome-obstruction of the SVC
- Horner syndrome-infiltration of cervical sympathetic chain by an apical tumor

Lung Cancer Review

Paraneoplastic Syndromes

- Pancoast syndrome-apical tumor infiltration of C8 and T1–T2
- Phrenic nerve palsy-tumor infiltration of phrenic nerve
- Recurrent laryngeal nerve palsy infiltration of recurrent laryngeal nerve
- Malignant pleural effusion-extension of tumor into the visceral and/or parietal pleura
- Hypertrophic pulmonary osteoarthropathy-periosteal proliferation of tubular bones
- Hypercalcemia-tumor secretes PTH analog (PTHrP), is secreted directly from tumor cells

Dx:
1. Physical exam
2. CXR
3. Obtain prior chest imaging if possible
4. Chest CT scan
5. Cytology of sputum-may diagnose central tumors (SCC tends to be central)
6. Whole body PET scan

Tx/Mgmt:
1. Referral to oncologist and surgical oncologist
2. Surgical/radiation/chemotherapy (not tested on Family Medicine Exam)

Adenocarcinoma of the Lung

Buzz Words: Persistent cough + hemoptysis + peripheral + osteoarthropathy + normal calcium level

Clinical Presentation: Similar to SCC of the lung, see above; however, adenocarcinoma tends to be found in more of a peripheral location, has higher incidence of hypertrophic pulmonary osteoarthropathy, and does not produce PTHrP. It is the most common primary lung malignancy in smokers and nonsmokers. Suspect adenocarcinoma when presenting symptoms are found in a nonsmoker.

PPx: (1) Smoking cessation, avoiding asbestos, and avoiding radon; (2) low-dose CT screening for those age 55–77 who have no symptoms and have a 30 pack-year smoking history (controversial)

MoD: (1) Malignant neoplastic gland formation possibly containing intracytoplasmic mucin

Dx: Same as lung SCC

Tx/Mgmt:
1. Referral to oncologist and surgical oncologist
2. Surgical/radiation/chemotherapy (not tested on Family Medicine Exam)

Small Cell Carcinoma of the Lung

Buzz Words: Smoker + persistent cough + hemoptysis + hyponatremia + Cushing's

Clinical Presentation: Similar to squamous cell carcinoma of the lung, see above; however, small cell carcinoma tends to be found more centrally and have different paraneoplastic syndromes. Paraneoplastic syndromes associated with small cell carcinoma include syndrome of inappropriate antidiuretic hormone secretion (SIADH), Cushing syndrome, and Eaton-Lambert syndrome.

PPx: (1) Smoking cessation, avoiding asbestos, and avoiding radon; (2) low-dose CT screening for those age 55–77 who have no symptoms and have a 30-pack per year smoking history (controversial)

MoD: Malignant, poorly differentiated small cells arising from neuroendocrine (Kulchitsky) cells. SIADH-ectopic secretion of ADH. Cushing syndrome-ectopic secretion of ACTH. Eaton-Lambert syndrome antibodies against presynaptic voltage-gated calcium channel leads to decreased release of acetylcholine.

Dx: Same as lung SCC

Tx/Mgmt:

1. Referral to oncologist and surgical oncologist
2. Surgical/radiation/chemotherapy (not tested on Family Medicine Exam) (Fig. 8.5)

Respiratory Failure/Respiratory Arrest and Pulmonary Vascular Disorders

Cardiogenic Pulmonary Edema

Buzz Words: Respiratory distress + crackles + history of orthopnea and/or paroxysmal nocturnal dyspnea (PND), S3 or S4, jugular venous distension (JVD)

Clinical Presentation: Dyspnea, hypoxemia, and crackles on lung auscultation. Patients may have tachycardia and hypertension. S3 or S4, JVD, and peripheral edema may also be present.

PPx: (1) Patient compliance: adherence to medications and dietary restrictions

MoD: Most often the result of acute decompensated heart failure (ADHF) due to ventricular systolic or diastolic dysfunction leading to a rapid and acute increase in left ventricular filling pressures and left atrial pressure. Ultimately this causes increased transudation of protein-poor fluid into the alveolar spaces. Causes of left ventricular systolic dysfunction include coronary heart disease,

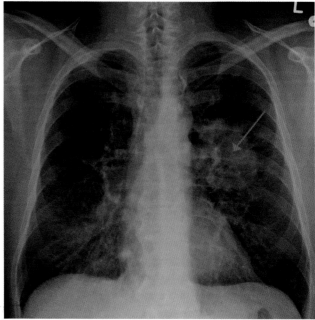

FIG. 8.5 X lung tumor (Wikipedia).

hypertension, valvular disease, and dilated cardiomyopathy. Causes of left ventricular diastolic dysfunction include hypertrophic and restrictive cardiomyopathies.

Dx:
1. Physical exam
2. CXR
3. ABG
4. ECG
5. Echocardiogram
6. Measure BNP

Tx/Mgmt:
1. Place patient sitting up with legs dangling from bed
2. Diuresis with daily assessment of weight,
3. Supplemental oxygen and assisted ventilation
4. Nitrates
5. Morphine

Pulmonary Embolism

Buzz Words: Dyspnea + chest pain + long periods of immobility

Clinical Presentation: The most common presenting symptom is dyspnea followed by pleuritic chest pain, cough, and symptoms of DVT. Rarely, as in the case of a massive PE, do patients present with hemoptysis, shock, syncope, and/or right bundle branch block. Many patients are asymptomatic or have mild symptoms. What is important to remember are the risk factors for PE. Inherited risk factors include factor V Leiden mutation, prothrombin gene mutation, protein S or C deficiency, and antithrombin deficiency. Acquired risk factors include malignancy, surgery (especially orthopedic procedures), trauma, prior DVT/PE, pregnancy, oral contraceptives, immobilization, congestive heart failure, obesity, and nephrotic syndrome.

PPx: Mobility after surgery or on airplanes

MoD: Virchow triad leads to a thrombus.

This thrombus, originating in another location of the body, embolizes to the pulmonary vasculature leading to three possible pathophysiologic responses: pulmonary infarction, abnormal gas exchange, and cardiovascular compromise. Pulmonary infarction is due to small thrombi travelling distally to the segmental and subsegmental vessels. Abnormal gas exchange is due to mechanical obstruction altering the ventilation-to-perfusion ratio, which creates dead space. Cardiovascular compromise is caused by increased pulmonary vascular resistance, which ultimately leads to an impeded right ventricular outflow and causes right heart strain.

QUICK TIPS

Virchow triad: venous stasis, endothelial injury, and hypercoagulable state

QUICK TIPS

Common sources of emboli include deep veins of the lower extremity (iliac, femoral, and popliteal) and deep veins of the pelvis.

Dx:

1. Physical exam
2. Use Modified Wells Criteria determined to determine likelihood of PE
3. D-dimer for unlikely probability of PE
4. Spiral CT for likely probability of PE
5. Leg ultrasound if spiral CT is inconclusive or cannot be performed
6. V/Q scan is reserved for those with suspected PE in whom spiral CT is contraindicated (renal insufficiency), inconclusive, or negative in the face of high clinical suspicion

gg AR

Well's Criteria for Pulmonary Embolism

gg AR

Algorithm for diagnosing PE

Tx/Mgmt:

1. Oxygen and fluids
2. Low-molecular-weight heparin (or unfractionated heparin)
3. Inferior vena cava (IVC) filter placement for those with contraindications to anticoagulation
4. Thrombolytic therapy, catheter-directed therapy, and/or thrombectomy for hemodynamically unstable patients
5. Long-term anticoagulation with factor Xa inhibitors (apixaban, edoxaban, rivaroxaban), direct thrombin inhibitors (dabigatran), or warfarin

Disorders of the Pleura, Mediastinum, and Chest Wall

Costochondritis

Buzz Words: Chest pain reproduced with palpation in young patient who thinks he or she has an MI

Clinical Presentation: Musculoskeletal chest pain often presents as an insidious and persistent pain. It can also be sharp and localized to a specific area. Pain is often reproducible upon palpation, which is key to differentiating costochondritis from other more serious causes of chest pain. The majority of chest wall pain associated with costochondritis is positional and will be exacerbated by deep breathing and movement. Patients will often not have the typical risk factors for cardiac causes of chest pain.

PPx: N/A

MoD: Inflammation of cartilage that connects ribs to sternum. Can be caused by physical strain, blow to the chest, arthritis, or joint infection.

Dx:
1. Physical exam
2. ECG
3. CXR

Tx/Mgmt:
1. Avoid strenuous activity
2. Stretching
3. Heat/cold packs
4. Over-the-counter NSAIDs

Spontaneous Pneumothorax

Buzz Words: Tall, lean, young men, acute respiratory distress

PPx: Smoking cessation

Clinical Presentation: Tachypnea, pleuritic chest pain, hypoxia, unilateral diminished or absent breath sounds, and unilateral hyperresonance to percussion. Primary spontaneous pneumothorax is more common in tall, lean, and young men and in smokers.

MoD: Pneumothorax is an abnormal collection of air in the pleural spaces that leads to an uncoupling of the lung from the chest wall. This leads to decreased lung volume and therefore hypoxia. Spontaneous pneumothorax may be classified as primary or secondary. Primary spontaneous pneumothorax occurs due to rupture of subpleural blebs without a precipitating event in a person who does not have lung disease. Secondary pneumothorax occurs in patients with underlying lung disease.

QUICK TIPS

Causes of secondary spontaneous pneumothorax: COPD, asthma, interstitial lung disease, neoplasm, cystic fibrosis, and tuberculosis

Dx:
1. Physical exam
2. CXR
3. Chest CT scan

Tx/Mgmt:
1. Supplemental oxygen if patient stable and small pneumothorax
2. Pleural aspiration if patient stable and large pneumothorax
3. Chest tube if clinical unstable pneumothorax
4. Pleurodesis via VATS for recurrent cases
5. Treat underlying illness

Traumatic Disorders of Upper Airways

Epistaxis

Buzz Words: Nosebleed, fall/winter season

PPx: No nose picking

Clinical Presentation: Patient presents with a nosebleed, a common occurrence that most patients do not seek care for.

MoD: Epistaxis can be broken down into two categories: anterior bleeds and posterior bleeds:

Anterior nosebleeds are often a result of mucosal trauma such as nose picking, but can also be due to low moisture. Posterior nosebleeds arise from the posterolateral branches of the sphenopalatine artery. Anterior and posterior nosebleeds may be associated with the following conditions: anticoagulation, hereditary hemorrhagic telangiectasia, platelet disorders, and aneurysm of the carotid artery.

Dx:
1. Physical exam
2. Coagulation study

Tx/Mgmt:
1. Self-resolve
2. Nasal packing
3. Balloon catheter for continuous posterior bleeding

> **QUICK TIPS**
>
> Anterior bleeds are by far the most common with 90% occurring within the vascular watershed area of the nasal septum known as Kiesselbach plexus.

Mechanical Disorders of the Upper and Lower Respiratory Tract

Obstructive Sleep Apnea

Buzz Words: Snoring, daytime somnolence, overweight

Clinical Presentation: Obstructive apneas, hypopneas, snoring, and resuscitative snorts. Daytime symptoms may include sleepiness, fatigue, or poor concentration.

Risk factors include advanced age, male gender, obesity, and craniofacial or upper airway soft tissue abnormalities.

PPx: (1) Weight loss

MoD: Recurrent, functional collapse during sleep of the velopharyngeal and/or oropharyngeal airway leading to reduced or complete cessation of airflow despite breathing efforts. Ultimately leads to hypercapnia and hypoxemia and fragmented sleep.

Dx:
1. In-laboratory polysomnography
2. Home sleep apnea testing

Tx/Mgmt:
1. Weight loss
2. CPAP
3. Oral appliances
4. Upper airway surgery to remove floppy tissue
5. Hypoglossal nerve stimulation

Central Sleep Apnea

Buzz Words: Cheyne-Stokes breathing, daytime somnolence, heart failure, stroke

Clinical Presentation: Symptoms of disrupted sleep, such as excessive daytime sleepiness, poor sleep quality, and poor concentration. May also present with PND, morning headaches, and nocturnal angina. Patients with heart failure or previous stroke are more likely to exhibit central sleep apnea with Cheyne-Stokes breathing.

Risk factors include advanced age, male sex, heart failure, stroke, and chronic opioid use.

PPx: N/A

MoD: Central nervous system fails to transmit proper signals to respiratory muscles. The most common type of central sleep apnea is due to hyperventilation: hypoxia (possibly due to secretions) triggers hyperpnea during sleep. This causes a ventilator overshoot leading to hypocapnia, which induces central apnea.

Dx: In-laboratory polysomnography

Tx/Mgmt:
1. CPAP
2. Adaptive servo-ventilation (ASC) for patients without heart failure
3. Nocturnal oxygen
4. Medical management of heart failure

Obesity-Hypoventilation Syndrome

Buzz Words: Symptoms of obstructive sleep apnea (OSA), signs of right-sided heart failure

Clinical Presentation: The majority of patients will have coexisting OSA and therefore the presentation is almost

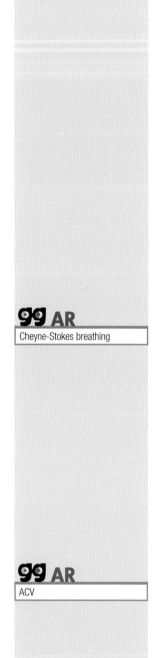

gg AR
Cheyne-Stokes breathing

gg AR
ACV

identical: obstructive apneas, hypopneas, snoring, and resuscitative snorts. Daytime symptoms may include sleepiness, fatigue, or poor concentration. Patients will often have severe obesity (BMI > 50 kg/m^2) and may have signs of right-sided heart failure.

PPx: Weight loss

MoD: The result of the complex interaction of several physiologic abnormalities such as sleep-disordered breathing (OSA), altered pulmonary function, and altered ventilatory control.

Dx:
1. Physical exam
2. ABG
3. Pulmonary function tests
4. Serum bicarbonate in-laboratory polysomnography
5. CXR

Tx/Mgmt:
1. Weight loss
2. CPAP
3. Abstain from alcohol and drugs that diminish respiratory drive such as benzodiazepines, opioids, and barbiturates

GUNNER PRACTICE

1. A 32-year-old man comes into your office with his wife because of fatigue during the daytime. He recently fell asleep at the wheel while driving and almost got into an accident. His physical exam is normal and his BMI is 32. His wife tells you he snores at night. Which of the following is the most appropriate next step in management?
   A. Weight loss
   B. CPAP
   C. Upper airway surgery
   D. Hypoglossal nerve stimulation
   E. Bariatric surgery

2. An 18-year-old comes to your practice complaining of recurrent episodes of shortness of breath and wheezing over the past month. On exam, his lungs are clear to auscultation and his physical exam is otherwise within normal limits. You diagnose him with asthma. Which of the following is the most appropriate pharmacologic intervention?
   A. Corticosteroids
   B. Albuterol
   C. Weight loss
   D. Ipatropium
   E. Watchful waiting

ANSWERS: What Would Gunner Jess/Jim Do?

1. **WWGJD?** A 32-year-old man comes into your office with his wife because of **fatigue during the daytime.** He recently fell asleep at the wheel while driving and almost got into an accident. His physical exam is normal and his **BMI is 32. His wife tells you he snores at night. Which of the following is the most appropriate next step in management?**

Answer: A. Weight loss. This is obstructive sleep apnea characterized by daytime fatigue, somnolence, and fatigue in the setting of someone who is both obese and snoring. First-line treatment is **always** weight loss.
   B. CPAP → This is not first-line treatment but would be the next step in management if weight loss fails.
   C. Upper airway surgery → This is a last resort treatment for OSA.
   D. Hypoglossal nerve stimulation → This is a last resort treatment for OSA.
   E. Bariatric surgery → This is a last resort treatment for morbid obesity (BMI > 40).

2. **WWGJD?** An 18-year-old comes to your practice complaining of recurrent episodes **of shortness of breath and wheezing over the past month.** On exam, his lungs are clear to auscultation and his physical exam is otherwise within normal limits. **You diagnose him with asthma. His episodes occur only once a week. Which of the following is the most appropriate pharmacologic intervention?**

Answer: B. Albuterol. Given the overall infrequency of his episodes, he should be started on a SABA for acute exacerbations in the form of an inhaler. This patient has intermittent asthma. Asthma is treated on the following basis:

Intermittent: symptoms ≤2 days/week
Nighttime awakenings ≤2×/month
SABA use ≤2 days/week
No interference with normal activity
Normal FEV1 between exacerbations, FEV1 greater than 80% predicted, FEV1/FVC normal
Step 1 treatment: SABA
Mild persistent: symptoms ≥2 days/week, but not daily
Nighttime awakenings 3–4≤ days/month
SABA use more than 2 days/week, but not daily; not more than once per day
Minor limitation with activity

Step 2 treatment: SABA + low-dose inhaled
  glucocorticoid
Moderate persistent: symptoms daily
Nighttime awakenings more than 1x/week, but not nightly
SABA use daily
Some limitation with activity
Step 3: SABA + low-dose inhaled glucocorticoid + LABA
Severe: symptoms throughout the day
Nighttime awakenings: nightly
SABA use several times per day
Extreme limitation of activity
Step 4: SABA + medium-dose inhaled glucocorticoid +
  LABA
Step 5: SABA + high-dose inhaled glucocorticoid + LABA
In severe cases, can move up to step 6 and add oral sys-
  temic glucocorticoids
  A. Corticosteroids → Incorrect. This is used to prevent
     recurrent asthma attacks for chronic asthmatics.
  C. Weight loss → Incorrect. There is no relationship
     between weight and asthma.
  D. Ipatropium → Incorrect. Often added to albuterol for
     more persistent asthma.
  E. Watchful waiting → Incorrect. Asthma will not tradi-
     tionally decline with age.

Nutritional and Digestive Disorders

Pujan Dave, Leo Wang, Hao-Hua Wu, and Judy Chertok

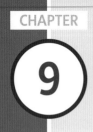

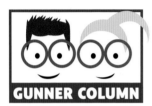

GUNNER COLUMN

Introduction

Diseases of the gastrointestinal (GI) system are often among the most challenging to master for many reasons. First, the breadth: the GI system spans from the lips and mouth down to the anus, and includes the pancreas, gallbladder, and liver. Second, the symptoms are often vague (e.g., abdominal pain, nausea) and overlap among the many pathologies. These problems are amplified in Family Medicine because of the broad age range of patients. This can make it difficult to pinpoint the underlying problem or the next step in management, especially in a multiple-choice question where you cannot ask the patients any additional questions.

To make this challenge more approachable, this chapter organizes the material in two ways. First, by general categorization: infectious, neoplastic, immune, ill-defined symptoms (e.g., nausea), and congenital. Second, the disorders are organized by anatomy (esophageal disorders, disorders of the stomach, etc.). This structure will highlight key differences between the presentations of different diseases and make it easier to choose the right answer in a multiple-choice question. The emphasis of the Family Medicine shelf exam is prevention/prophylaxis, and so it is important to take note of these as you read.

About 5%–10% of the Family Medicine shelf exam will focus on nutritional and digestive disorders. However, since the GI system is so systemically involved, having GI symptoms does not necessarily mean that they have a primary GI illness. Thus, it is important to approach each question holistically and keep an eye out for Buzz Words or diagnostic studies that can point you in the right direction.

Infectious Disorders

Bacterial

Staphylococcus aureus

Buzz Words: N/V + abdominal pain + recent ingestion of dairy product (e.g., old mayonnaise)

Clinical Presentation: Fast onset (1–6 hours) food poisoning; nausea, vomiting, abdominal cramps

PPx: (1) Adequate refrigeration of food products. (2) Hand hygiene.

MoD: Heat-stable enterotoxin B acts as a superantigen by forming a bridge between MHC-II on antigen presenting cells and T-cell receptors on T-cells.

Dx:

1. Clinical diagnosis
2. Vomitus and/or food can be tested for the enterotoxin

Tx/Mgmt: Self-limited, offer supportive therapy

Escherichia coli

Buzz Words: Hemolytic uremic syndrome (HUS) + schistocytes + hemorrhagic diarrhea + recently ate undercooked meat (e.g., hamburgers) → Enterohemorrhagic *E. coli* (EHEC)

Clinical Presentation:

There are four types of *E. coli* that can be tested by the NBME (see below). Of the four, EHEC is the most high yield. If pressed for time, skip EPEC, ETEC, and EIEC:

1. Enterohemorrhagic *E. coli* (EHEC)—Shiga-like toxin from undercooked meat leading to HUS. Most commonly tested. Make sure to learn how to identify this one only.
2. Enteropathogenic *E. coli* (EPEC)—Predominates in children (peds), non-bloody diarrhea.
3. Enterotoxifenic *E. coli* (ETEC)—Travelers' diarrhea, nonbloody diarrhea, second most commonly tested.
4. Enteroinvasive *E. coli* (EIEC)—Inflammatory bowel, bloody diarrhea.

PPx: (1) Hand washing. (2) Adequate sanitization of water. (3) Avoiding food contamination.

ETEC causes secretory diarrhea. Patients traveling to endemic areas can take antibiotics (fluoroquinolones first-line, azithromycin if going to Asia) and use them in case of developing diarrhea during their trip; these decrease the duration of symptoms.

MoD:

For EHEC: Shiga toxin (verotoxin) → inactivates ribosomal 60S component → endothelial damage (gut, kidney, lung) → hemorrhage:

- no need to know MoD of ETEC, EIEC, or EPEC for the shelf

> **QUICK TIPS**
>
> Triad of HUS: anemia + thrombocytopenia + acute kidney injury (AKI)

- only thing that is pertinent is that EHEC and EIEC →
  bloody diarrhea = bacteria invade mucosa
- ETEC and EPEC do not invade and inflame gut
  mucosa

Dx:

1. Blood culture and Gram stain (motile, encapsulated
   Gram-negative rod, catalase [+], and oxidase [–])
2. MacConkey agar (pink; lactose fermenter)
3. DNA assays, enzyme immunoassays for toxin
4. For EHEC, complete blood count (CBC), BMP

Tx/Mgmt:

1. Supportive therapy (i.e., fluids)
2. Avoid antiperistaltic agents (loperamide) as these
   might prolong the duration of infection
3. For EHEC
   a. fluid replacement
   b. avoid antibiotics, which may precipitate HUS
      (Table 9.1)

Listeria monocytogenes

Buzz Words: Pasteurized milk + dark/cloudy amniotic fluid +
newborn meningitis → *Listeria*

Clinical Presentation: Febrile gastroenteritis which might
progress to systemic disease in pregnant patients, during steroid therapy, or in the immunosuppressed. *Listeria*
is also the third most common cause of meningitis in
newborns and is the reason why **ampicillin** is added to
the treatment regimen at times with ≤6-month-old
infants with sepsis.

TABLE 9.1 Most Common Diarrheal Illnesses Caused by *E. coli*

	ETEC (i.e., Traveler's Diarrhea)	EHEC (*O157:H7 Serotype*)	EIEC
Presentation	Watery diarrhea	Hemorrhagic colitis and HUS in 8% of cases	Dysentery 12–72 h after ingestion
MoD	Heat-labile toxin (LT) and heat-stable toxin (ST) activate adenylate and guanylate cyclase respec- tively → secretory diarrhea	Shiga toxin (verotoxin) → inactivates ribosomal 60S component → endo- thelial damage (gut, kid- ney, lung) → hemorrhage	Mucosal cell invasion causing membrane disruption
Clinical cues	Traveler's and children <5 years old	Children and elderly; trans- mitted through under- cooked ground beef	Developing countries; invasion rarely goes beyond submucosa
Management	Fluid replacement Ciprofloxacin	Fluid replacement; avoid antibiotics! These may precipitate HUS	Fluid replacement

EHEC, Enterohemorrhagic *E. coli; EIEC,* enteroinvasive *E. coli; ETEC,* enterotoxifenic *E. coli; HUS,* hemolytic uremic
syndrome; *LT,* heat-labile toxin; *ST,* heat-stable toxin.

PPx: N/A

MoD:

1. Motile by actin filament polymerization
2. Transmitted through contaminated dairy products and deli meat. The organism can survive refrigerator temperatures and a wide range of pH.

Dx: Stool culture and Gram stain (shows tumbling motility; catalase [+], Gram-positive; facultative anaerobe).

Tx/Mgmt:

1. Ampicillin
2. TMP/SMX (antibiotic resistance is rare)

Yersinia enterocolitica

Buzz Words: Diarrhea + young patient + pharyngitis + mesenteric lymphadenitis

Clinical Presentation: Enterocolitis in children may be accompanied by pharyngitis (no other cause of bacterial diarrhea). Mesenteric lymphadenitis that simulates acute appendicitis. Associated with HLA-B27 tissue type (seronegative spondyloarthropathies), may have erythema nodosum and reactive arthritis as sequelae.

PPx: (1) Avoid contact with canine feces and hand washing after exposure to swine products.

MoD: Organism courses through the stomach, attaches and invades the gut wall to end up localizing in regional lymphoid tissue.

Dx: Culture isolation from stool, pharynx, or mesenteric nodes

Tx/Mgmt: Ciprofloxacin (adults) or TMP-SMX (children) only in patients with severe disease only

Campylobacter spp.

Buzz Words: Bloody diarrhea + fever + cramping periumbilical abdominal pain

Clinical Presentation: Bloody diarrhea, fever, and cramping periumbilical abdominal pain. Children may manifest abdominal pain that mimics appendicitis or colitis. Guillain-Barré syndrome (ascending paralysis), HUS, and reactive arthritis are late onset complications.

PPx: (1) Avoid eating raw/undercooked meat.

MoD: Invasive with a low infective dose (~500 bacteria). Poultry reservoir. Puppies are the most common source of infection for children. Produces crypt abscesses resembling ulcerative colitis. Disease is self-limited with a mean duration of 7 days.

Dx:

1. Stool culture
2. Serologic test may be used to detect recent infection once the organism is no longer in the stool

Tx/Mgmt:

1. Supportive therapy
2. Fluoroquinolones, azithromycin, or erythromycin in setting of severe diarrhea

Salmonella spp.

Buzz Words: Fever + abdominal cramps + diarrhea + chicken + fever + 60% lymphs

Sickle cell patient + osteomyelitis → *Salmonella* infx

Clinical Presentation: Inflammatory diarrhea, nausea, vomit, fever, and abdominal cramps; important cause of osteomyelitis in patients with sickle cell disease

PPx: (1) Adequate hygiene. (2) Live-attenuated (Ty21a) or Vi capsular vaccines exist.

MoD: Transmitted through ingestion of poultry, eggs, and milk products. The organism invades the intestinal wall and submucosal lymphoid system, to the circulation, and finally finds shelter within macrophages of the reticuloendothelial system. Type III secretion system and lipid A are the two main virulence factors. Chronic carriage state (>1 year) most usually occurs in elderly patients with biliary tract abnormalities (gallstones most commonly).

Dx: Stool culture (H2S [+], motile, acid-labile, capsulated, Gram-negative bacilli, black colonies on Hektoen agar, pea-soup diarrhea).

Tx/Mgmt:

1. Supportive therapy
2. Antibiotic therapy (fluoroquinolones) is only warranted for severe infection or patients with risk factors

Shigella spp.

Buzz Words: Bloody diarrhea + day-care center, mental institution + beef ingestion

Clinical Presentation: Patient has frequent, small volume, bloody stools with fever, abdominal cramps, and tenesmus. Intestinal complications involve toxic megacolon, colonic perforation, intestinal obstruction, proctitis, and rectal prolapse. Thrombocytopenia and HUS are common in young children (similar to EHEC); other systemic complications include protein-loss enteropathy, leukemoid reaction, neurological manifestation, and reactive arthritis.

PPx: (1) Adequate hygiene

MoD: Invasion of M cells. Toxin inactivates ribosomal 60S subunit (similar to verotoxin in EHEC). Glomerular damage. Spreads fecal–oral, hand–hand.

Dx: Stool culture to isolate bacteria (acid-stable, immotile, Gram-negative bacilli; green colonies on Hektoen agar)

Tx/Mgmt:

1. Supportive therapy; self-limited infection
2. Antibiotics (ceftriaxone or azithromycin) are appropriate for children and immunosuppressed patients

Viral

Non-polio Enterovirus Enteritis/Colitis (Echovirus, Coxsackievirus)

Buzz Words: Abdominal pain + watery diarrhea + sick contact

Clinical Presentation: Frequently asymptomatic or presents as an undifferentiated febrile illness. If GI symptoms are present, may produce a mild watery diarrhea. More common in children.

PPx: N/A

MoD: Virus replicates in the pharynx and intestines and is secreted in stool (person-to-person, fecal-oral spread)

Dx:

1. Clinical diagnosis of acute gastroenteritis
2. Laboratory studies not needed

Tx/Mgmt:

1. Symptom management
2. Rehydration
3. If suspect non-polio enterovirus, be watchful for non-gastrointestinal viral exanthems, such as aseptic meningitis, encephalitis, myocarditis, petechiae/purpura, and others

Parasitic

Giardia

Buzz Words: Camping + drink water from outdoor source + foul-smelling stools

Clinical Presentation: Classically, a profuse, watery diarrhea with foul-smelling stools associated with bloating, flatulence, abdominal cramps, and malaise in the acute setting. Malabsorption can lead to weight loss, hypoalbuminemia, and vitamin deficiencies. Symptoms last for 2–4 weeks, but half of patients develop chronic, intermittent symptoms. Increased risk in patients with B-cell disorders such as immunoglobulin (Ig)A deficiency.

PPx: (1) Handwashing. (2) Effective water sanitation.

MoD: *Giardia* primarily infects the small intestine and causes increased permeability and decreased absorption due to reduction of brush border enzymes (e.g., lactase).

Dx:
1. Antigen detection assay of stool (ELISA)
2. Nucleic acid amplification assays (NAAT) of stool
3. Stool microscopy (least preferred) showing multinucle-ated, pear-shaped trophozoites with multiple flagella or oval, multinucleated cysts.

Tx/Mgmt:
1. Metronidazole
2. Supportive care (rehydration)

Immunologic and Inflammatory Disorders

Celiac Disease

Buzz Words: Flattened villi + chronic diarrhea with exposure to gluten

Clinical Presentation: Symptoms of malabsorption. Chronic diarrhea and abdominal pain. May have skin lesions (dermatitis herpetiformis). Associated with other autoimmune conditions.

PPx: Gluten-free diet (avoid wheat, barley, and rye)

MoD: Autoimmune (T-cell and IgA-mediated response) against a breakdown product of gluten.

Dx:
1. Anti-tissue transglutaminase and anti-endomysial antibodies are the most diagnostic
2. Anti-gliadin antibodies may be elevated
3. GD/colonoscopy biopsies will show atrophy of the villi, crypt hyperplasia, and intraepithelial lymphocytosis.

Tx/Mgmt: Gluten-free diet

Inflammatory Bowel Disease

Inflammatory bowel disease (IBD) is commonly thought of as an inpatient disease, since exacerbations of IBD are often treated in the hospital. For the purposes of the Family Medicine exam, Tx/Mgmt is low-yield. Focus on the PPx, especially with regard to colon cancer screening guidelines

According to the American Cancer Society (ACS), colon cancer screening in IBD patients should be a colonoscopy every 1 or 2 years starting 8 years after disease onset.

Crohn Disease

Buzz Words: Bloody diarrhea + skip lesions on colonoscopy + string-sign on barium swallow

Clinical Presentation: Non-specific and varied. Presents with diarrhea (may be bloody), weight loss, and abdominal pain. Patients may have rash (erythema nodosum, pyoderma gangrenosum), joint pain, aphthous ulcers, or eye pain (uveitis). Notably, patients may have fistulas, fissures, and abscesses.

PPx: (1) ACS guidelines from screening for colon cancer. (2) Avoid smoking.

MoD: Transmural inflammation anywhere along the GI tract, except the rectum. Most common location is the terminal ileum.

Dx:
1. CBC (elevated white blood count and anemia)
2. ESR/CRP (elevated)
3. EGD/colonoscopy

Tx/Mgmt:
1. Steroids
2. Disease modifying anti-rheumatologic agents (e.g., methotrexate)
3. Biologics (e.g., anti-tumor necrosis factor [TNF] alpha inhibitors)

Ulcerative Colitis

Buzz Words: Bloody diarrhea + primary sclerosing cholangitis + only involvement in colon

Clinical Presentation: Presents with bloody diarrhea, abdominal pain, tenesmus, and rectal urgency. Patients may have rash (erythema nodosum, pyoderma gangrenosum), joint pain, aphthous ulcers, or eye pain (uveitis). Increased risk for colon cancer. Major complication is toxic megacolon.

PPx: (1) ACS guidelines from screening for colon cancer. (2) Avoid smoking.

MoD:
Continuous circumferential mucosal inflammation that begins in the rectum.

Dx:
1. CBC (elevated white blood count and anemia)
2. ESR/CRP (elevated)
3. EGD/colonoscopy

Tx/Mgmt:
1. Steroids
2. Disease-modifying anti-rheumatologic agents (e.g., 5-ASA, methotrexate)
3. Biologics (e.g., anti-TNF alpha inhibitors)
4. Surgery

Neoplasms

Colon Polyps
Buzz Words: Melana + >50-year-old patient

Clinical Presentation: Most commonly discovered in patients >50 years old on screening colonoscopy, but may also be found on barium enema or computed tomography (CT) scan. Polyps are typically asymptomatic but some may ulcerate and cause gross or occult bleeding. On colonoscopy, polyps are characterized as flat, sessile, or pedunculated. Polyps may be neoplastic or non-neoplastic, depending on its histologic type. Hyperplastic (most common), mucosal, and hamartomatous polyps are non-neoplastic. Adenomatous and serrated polyps can be cancerous or precancerous.

PPx: (1) Starting at age 50, colonoscopy every 10 years until 75 (76–85 on an individual basis).

MoD: Varies based on histologic type, but typically involves specific mutations (in APC or KRAS genes) or epigenetic changes (CpG hypermethylation, for example).

Dx: Colonoscopy is the gold standard for diagnosis.

Tx/Mgmt:

1. Polypectomy during colonoscopy for complete removal of the polyp
2. Follow-up colonoscopy based on age of patient, type of polyps, and number of polyps

Signs, Symptoms, and Ill-Defined Disorders

The purpose of this subsection is to illustrate common chief complaints you may encounter on the Family Medicine exam and potential etiologies.

Upper Gastrointestinal Bleeding

Buzz Words: Melena, hematemesis

Clinical Presentation: Hematemesis (bright red or coffee ground), epigastric pain, and/or melena. May present with hematochezia if bleed is brisk. Not all dark stool is melena; certain foods (spinach) and medications (iron pills, charcoal, licorice) can darken stool. Exam may be positive for orthostasis or other signs of volume depletion. Rectal exam may show hemoccult positive stools. Labs may be consistent with iron-deficiency anemia due to blood loss.

PPx: (1) Depends on underlying condition (e.g., proton pump inhibitor (PPI) use for patients with peptic ulcer disease (PUD), non-selective beta-blocker for esophageal varices, etc.).

MoD: Bleeding that originates from a source above the ligament of Treitz. Etiologies include:
Oropharyngeal bleeding
Epistaxis

Mallory-Weiss tear

Vascular lesions (dieulafoy's, AVM, gastric antral vascular ectasia [GAVE])

Erosive esophagitis

PUD

Neoplasm

Varices

Dx:

1. History and physical exam
2. Nasogastric (NG) tube lavage can help determine upper versus lower GI source, but may not be accurate if the bleeding is not constant in an upper source
3. Upper endoscopy once patient is stable (diagnostic and therapeutic intervention).

Tx/Mgmt:

1. First, assess severity and resuscitate to hemodynamic stability (ABCs, two large-bore [16- or 18-gauge] IVs, IVF or blood products as needed, supplemental oxygen, reverse any coagulopathies)
2. Labs: CBC, comprehensive metabolic panel (CMP), coagulation studies, type & screen (or cross, depending on clinical context). Monitor labs as frequently as clinically indicated
3. Start PPI
4. Upper endoscopy for diagnosis and therapeutic intervention once stable
5. Surgery if hemodynamically unstable despite above interventions, persistent bleeding for over 24 hours, or recurrence of bleed/high chance of recurrence

Lower Gastrointestinal Bleeding (Hematochezia, BRBPR)

Buzz Words: Loose maroon stools + bright red blood per rectum

Clinical Presentation: Bright red blood per rectum, hematochezia, loose, maroon stools (blood is a cathartic) with blood clots, and tenesmus. Exam may be positive for orthostasis or other signs of volume depletion. Rectal exam may show hemoccult positive stools. Labs may be consistent with iron deficiency anemia due to blood loss.

PPx: (1) Depends on underlying condition

MoD: Bleeding that originates below the ligaments of Treitz. Etiologies include:

Hemorrhoids

Anal fissures

PUD

Diverticulosis

Vascular lesions (AVM, angiodysplasia, etc.)

IBD

Polyp

Neoplasia

Ischemic colitis

Mesenteric ischemia

Dx:

1. History and physical exam
2. NG tube lavage can help determine upper versus lower GI source
3. Colonoscopy once patient is stable (diagnostic and therapeutic intervention)
4. Tagged RBC scan (radionuclide scan) to identify active bleeding
5. Angiography (requires active bleeding, can be therapeutic with embolization or medication administration)
6. CT angiogram (check renal function before giving contrast)
7. Capsule endoscopy or push enteroscopy if suspicious for small intestinal source.

Tx/Mgmt:

1. First, assess severity and resuscitate to hemodynamic stability (ABCs, two large-bore [16- or 18-gauge] IVs, IVF or blood products as needed, supplemental oxygen, reverse coagulopathies)
2. Labs: CBC, CMP, coagulation studies, type & screen (or cross, depending on clinical context). Monitor labs as frequently as clinically indicated
3. Colonoscopy for diagnosis and therapeutic intervention once stable
4. Surgery if hemodynamically unstable despite above interventions, persistent bleeding for over 24 hours, or recurrence of bleed/high chance of recurrence.

Constipation

Buzz Words: Pain with defecation + difficulty producing bowel movements

Clinical Presentation: Patients who are constipated have less than three bowel movements (BMs) in 1 week. There is also history of straining, reduced stool frequency, hard stools, incomplete movements, or sensation of obstruction. May also have vague abdominal pain, bloating, or encoparesis. Important to watch for "alarm" symptoms (weight loss, fevers, anorexia, blood in stools, or family history of IBD).

Rome criteria for constipation

PPx: (1) High-fiber diet, maintaining hydration and drinking enough fluids. (2) Avoid opiates and other medications that increase risk.

MoD: Some etiologies include:

1. Functional (slow transit, pelvic floor dysfunction, irritable bowel syndrome [IBS])
2. Medication (narcotic analgesics including opioids, chronic laxative abuse, anticholinergic, CCB)
3. Metabolic (hypothyroid, uremia, dehydration, hypokalemia, hypomagnesemia, hypercalcemia)
4. Obstruction (hernia, mass/cancer, CF)
5. Neurogenic (DM gastroparesis or enteropathy, PD, Hirschsprung, scleroderma-related, amyloid), ileus, or extreme dyschezia

Dx:

1. Important to rule out obstruction with history and physical (including DRE). If concerned, obtain abdominal plain film
2. Labs: CBC, TSH, electrolyte levels
3. Colonoscopy or flexible sigmoidoscopy if there are "alarm" symptoms.

Tx/Mgmt:

1. Diet and behavioral modification. The three Fs: increase Fluids, increase Fiber, and increase "F"ysical activity
2. In the acute setting, try a bulking agent (psyllium, fiber, etc.), followed by an osmotic laxative (lactulose, polyethylene glycol, etc.), followed by a secretory laxative (bisacodyl, etc.)
3. Enema (fleet [unless chronic kidney disease or ESRD], tap water, SMOG) if the above is not successful.

Diarrhea

Buzz Words: At least three loose BMs per day

Clinical Presentation: Increased stool frequency. Acute if less than 2–4 weeks, otherwise chronic. May be watery, bloody, greasy, or foul-smelling. Patients may also have fever, rash, abdominal pain, nausea, vomiting, tenesmus, dyschezia, urgency, or volume depletion, depending on the underlying etiology. Sometimes, the underlying cause of loose stools is actually constipation with stool maneuvering around a fecal impaction. It is important to note any history of immunocompromise (see infection section above).

PPx: (1) Depends on underlying etiology

MoD: In the acute setting:

Infectious

Medications (e.g., laxatives)

Malabsorption

Ischemic bowel

Intestinal tumors

Chronic causes include:

Motility dysfunction (IBS, scleroderma)

Medications (PPI, selective serotonin reuptake inhibitor [SSRI], non-steroidal anti-inflammatory drugs [NSAIDs])

Malabsorption (pancreatic insufficiency, celiac)

Inflammation (IBD, infection, radiation)

Osmotic (lactose intolerance)

Secretory

Dx:

1. History and physical exam (including DRE)
2. If chronic, bloody, dehydration, immunodeficiency, or suspicion for IBD, obtain CBC, stool sample (fecal leukocytes, ova and parasites, culture, calprotectin or lactoferrin, *Clostridium difficile* toxin polymerase chain reaction [if recent hospitalization or antibiotics])
3. Flexible sigmoidoscopy or colonoscopy if chronic without a clear cause
4. Other specific tests as needed depending on clinical situation (e.g., hydrogen breath test for lactose intolerance)

Tx/Mgmt:

1. Supportive treatment with oral rehydration therapy. Can be done in the outpatient setting for most cases. If the patient cannot tolerate PO, has profuse bloody diarrhea, or is toxic-appearing, admit for IVF and further management
2. Do not start give an anti-motility agent (loperamide) in the concern about an inflammatory or infectious cause due to increased risk of toxic megacolon
3. Empiric antibiotics if concerned for bacterial etiology (e.g., ciprofloxacin ± metronidazole)
4. Use ciprofloxacin for traveler's diarrhea

Disorders of the Upper Gastrointestinal Tract

Achalasia

Buzz Words: Barium swallow showing dilated esophagus with "bird beak sign"

Clinical Presentation: Presents with non-progressive solid and liquid dysphagia and burning chest pain (may complain of "heartburn" that does not respond to PPI therapy). Patients may also regurgitate food.

PPx: N/A

MoD: Inability of LES to relax due to degeneration of Auerbach ganglion cells. Most often idiopathic, but may be infectious (Chagas) or pseudoachalasia (tumor at the LES).

Dx:

1. Barium swallow (bird's beak narrowing of the distal esophagus)
2. Manometry (elevated LES pressure)
3. Esophagogastroduodenoscopy ([EGD]; difficult to pass scope into the stomach)

Tx/Mgmt:

1. Pneumatic dilation during EGD
2. Surgical management is myotomy (laparoscopic or new Per Oral Endoscopic Myotomy [POEM]).

Zenker Diverticulum

Buzz Words: Malodorous breath

Clinical Presentation: Elderly male with dysphagia, regurgitation of food, and halitosis

PPx: N/A

MoD: False diverticulum that forms due to esophageal dysmotility.

Dx: Barium swallow is diagnostic (first cup will fall and rest in the diverticulum). Do not pass an NG tube due to risk of perforation.

Tx/Mgmt: Endoscopic or surgical treatment

Gastroesophageal Reflux Disease

Buzz Words: Nocturnal dry cough + adult-onset asthma

Clinical Presentation: Very high yield. Presents with chronic cough, dysphagia, chest pain (retrosternal heartburn-like), and food regurgitation. Exacerbated when lying down. Associated with sliding hiatal hernias (type 1 esophageal hiatal hernia).

PPx: (1) Avoid eating while lying down, caffeine, alcohol, smoking, spicy foods, fatty foods, carbonated beverages, and peppermint from the diet. (2) Weight loss may also help.

MoD: Inappropriately relaxed LES (opposite of achalasia) that allows food in the stomach to travel back up the esophagus.

Dx: Clinical picture and improvement of symptoms with PPI

Tx/Mgmt:

1. Lifestyle modification
2. PPI effective but risk factors associated with long-term use
3. Surgery is last resort (Nissen fundoplication)

Peptic Ulcer Disease (Gastric Ulcer, Duodenal Ulcer)

Buzz Words: Chronic musculoskeletal pain (insinuates long-term daily use of NSAIDs)

Clinical Presentation: Aching epigastric/right upper quadrant pain, nausea, vomiting, and bloating, but may be painless especially if using NSAIDs. Pain immediately after meals favors gastric ulcer, while pain relief with meals favors duodenal ulcer. Patients often have a history of NSAID use for musculoskeletal pain. Complications include hemorrhage (most common complication), obstruction, and perforation. Perforation is a surgical emergency that presents with fever, leukocytosis, shoulder pain (referred), free air under the diaphragm on X-ray, and wall thickening with fluid collection on CT scan.

PPx: Avoidance of NSAIDs or use NSAID with misoprostol

MoD: Disruption of mucosal barrier leading to a defect in the gastric or duodenal wall down to the muscularis mucosa (beyond muscularis is a perforation). Etiologies include NSAID use, *Helicobacter pylori* infection, ZES, and smoking.

Dx:
1. Upper endoscopy with biopsy is the gold standard and is required to rule out gastric malignancy
2. Serum gastrin levels if suspicious for ZES
3. *H. pylori* can be diagnosed with biopsy, serum antibody, stool testing, and urea breath testing.

Tx/Mgmt:
1. Acid suppression (H2 blocker, PPI, antacid)
2. Avoid NSAID/aspirin use or use NSAID with misoprostol
3. Smoking cessation and reduce alcohol use
4. Avoid eating close to bedtime
5. Triple or quadruple for *H. pylori* (PPI + amoxicillin + clarithromycin, or PPI + amoxicillin + clarithromycin + bismuth subsalicylate)
6. Surgery for perforation

Gastroparesis

Buzz Words: Delay in emptying of stomach

Clinical Presentation: Diabetic patient with constipation, nausea, bloating, post-prandial fullness, and vague abdominal discomfort or pain.

PPx: Proper management of underlying diseases

MoD: Disruption of the autonomic nervous system (afferent gastric nerves, i.e., from prolonged hyperglycemia). Most common causes include diabetes, post-surgical, and idiopathic (often post-viral). Could also be medication-induced.

Dx: Clinical diagnosis. If concerning features, rule out gastric outlet obstruction with imaging (UGI series or CT) or EGD and obtain gastric emptying scan (solid-phase, i.e., barium-soaked bread).

Tx/Mgmt:
1. Dietary modification (avoid fatty, acidic, high-fiber foods)
2. Metoclopramide (long-term use can cause tardive dyskinesia!)
3. Macrolide antibiotics (promote gastric motility)
4. Optimize glycemic control
5. Surgery if refractory to medical management

Disorders of the Small Intestine, Colon, Rectum, and Anus

Irritable Bowel Syndrome

Buzz Words: Abdominal pain relieved with bowel movement, alternating constipation and diarrhea

Clinical Presentation: Woman with non-specific abdominal pain and/or alternating constipation and diarrhea. Pain triggered by stress. Pain relieved with bowel movements. No nocturnal symptoms. Four subtypes: predominant diarrhea, constipation, mixed, and post-viral.

PPx: Dietary modification (FODMAPs diet, discussed below)

MoD: Decreased serotonin metabolism (altered gut motility, visceral hypersensitivity) and genetic component.

Dx:
1. Follows specific Rome IV criteria (pain at least once a week for 3 months, associated with defecation or change in bowel frequency or consistency).
2. Exclude other pathologies based on symptoms such as IBD and celiac.

Tx/Mgmt:
Treatment depends on subtype.
1. Constipation predominant is treated with high fiber diet, laxative, lubiprostine, or linaclotide.
2. Diarrhea predominant is treated with loperamide or certain anticholinergics.
3. Pain managed with SSRI or low dose TCA.
4. FODMAPs (fermentable oligo-, di-, and monosaccharides and polyols) diet is perhaps the most effective.

Lactose Intolerance

Buzz Words: Diarrhea after ingestion of dairy

Clinical Presentation: Presents with diarrhea, bloating, and flatulence after ingesting milk products

PPx: (1) Avoid lactose-containing products.

MoD: Deficiency of lactase, which metabolizes lactose that is found in dairy products, (i.e., post-gastroenteritis) enables milk to pass undigested into the distal small bowel and colon.

Dx: Clinical history and improvement with avoiding ingesting dairy products. Can also use hydrogen breath test, stool pH (<6.0), and stool osmotic gap (>125 mOsm/kg).

Tx/Mgmt: Avoidance of milk and lactase supplementation

Perirectal/Perianal Abscess

Buzz Words: (1) Fluctuant mass at the anal verge

Clinical Presentation: Severe anal pain, fever, and malaise. Exam may show mass or indurated area in the perianal or perirectal region. Associated with pilonidal cysts and Crohn disease.

PPx: N/A

MoD: Obstruction of perianal crypt glands that results in infection

Dx: Clinical diagnosis. However, if abscess cannot be confirmed on exam, do imaging (CT or magnetic resonance imaging).

Tx/Mgmt: Incision and drainage

Anal Fissure

Buzz Words: Blood-streaked stool or blood on toilet paper + Crohn disease

Clinical Presentation: Female patient with severe, localized, tearing anal pain with bowel movements. Stool may be blood streaked or may find blood when wiping with tissue paper.

PPx: (1) Avoid hard stools (high fiber diet, fluids, etc.). (2) Reinforce proper anal hygiene. (3) Keep anal area dry. (4) Avoid straining during defecation.

MoD: Linear tear in the rectal canal, usually in the posterior region. Etiology is a tight anal sphincter. Associated with Crohn disease.

Dx: Physical exam shows fissure. However, patients are in extreme pain and may be difficult to examine without sedation.

Tx/Mgmt:

1. Sitz bath, increase dietary fiber, and local analgesics for pain.
2. Topical vasodilators such as nifedipine, diltiazem, or nitroglycerin can be used with stool softeners and laxatives.
3. Surgery for refractory cases.

Hemorrhoids

Buzz Words: Rectal mass + blood on tissue paper

Clinical Presentation: Anal pain, pruritus, and blood on tissue paper or feces. Hemorrhoids may be internal (proximal to dentate line, usually painless) or external hemorrhoids (distal to dentate line, usually painful).

PPx: Prevent constipation (high-fiber diet, adequate fluid intake, etc.)

MoD: Distension of venous plexus from deterioration of connective tissue that anchors the hemorrhoid and increased anal tone

Dx:
1. Physical exam
2. Anoscopy

Tx/Mgmt:
1. Avoid constipation and straining, as above
2. Hydrocortisone cream or suppositories with warm sitz baths
3. Medicated wipes such as Tucks wipes
4. Topical analgesics for pain control
4. Last resort is surgery

Disorders of the Liver and Biliary System

Bile Duct Obstruction/Cholestasis

Buzz Words: Jaundice + pruritus + pale colored stools + dark-colored urine

Clinical Presentation: Patients present acutely with jaundice, pale-colored stools, and dark-colored urine. Other symptoms include diarrhea due to malabsorption and pruritus from increased bile acids in the blood. Cholestasis may be due to intrahepatic or extrahepatic obstruction.

PPx: N/A

MoD: Intrahepatic or extrahepatic obstruction. Can be due to hepatitis, medication use (OCP, anabolic steroids), pregnancy (estrogen inhibits bile acid secretion), physical obstruction (tumor, stone, etc.) and metabolic disorders.

Dx:
1. Hyperbilirubinemia (majority conjugated), hypercholesterolemia, bilirubinuria, absence of urobilinogen in urine.
2. Alk phos and GGT are elevated more than AST/ALT.

Tx/Mgmt:
1. Treatment is based on underlying cause.
2. Ursodeoxycholic acid is can be used to improve bile flow and treat pruritus.

Cholelithiasis (Gallstones)

Buzz Words: Abdominal pain + right shoulder pain, post-prandial pain, four Fs (fat, female, forty, fertile)

Clinical Presentation: Often asymptomatic or an incidental finding on imaging in a female in her 40s who has a history of OCP use. Symptoms may include abdominal pain with shoulder pain (Boas sign) and post-prandial pain. Risk factors include fibrates, female sex, OCPs, obesity, Crohn disease, cirrhosis, hemolytic anemia, TPN, and helminth biliary tract infection. Complications include bile duct obstruction, gallstone ileus, choledo-cholithiasis, and cholecystitis, pancreatitis.

PPx: (1) Weight loss. Avoid precipitating medications in patients with multiple risk factors.

MoD: (1) Supersaturation of bilirubin or cholesterol. (2) Decreased bile salts/acids or phospholipids in bile. (3) Cholesterol stones are the most common (IBD, obesity, age, estrogen, pregnancy, rapid weight loss). (4) Pigment stones are seen with chronic hemolysis (e.g., thalassemia, sickle cell, etc.), cirrhosis, and TPN.

Dx: Ultrasound shows echogenic foci in the gallbladder.

Tx/Mgmt: Prophylactic cholecystectomy if symptomatic or at an increased risk for gallbladder cancer.

GUNNER PRACTICE

1. A 10-month-old male is brought in by his mother for decreased energy and worsening instability while crawling or walking for the past several weeks. According to the mother, this patient was "yellow" shortly after birth and had dark urine and pale stools. He required a GI procedure at 1 month of age. Since then, the patient has been awaiting a liver transplant. The patient does not take any medications or supplements. On exam, the patient has normal morphologic features, sub-lingual jaundice, and pale conjunctiva. Laboratory results are notable for unconjugated hyperbilirubinemia, decreased haptoglobin, elevated LDH, decreased hemoglobin, elevated ALP, and elevated AST/ALT. Anti-smooth muscle antibody (ASMA), anti-nuclear antibody (ANA), anti-liver kidney microsomal antibodies (anti-LKM), and anti-soluble liver antigen (SLA) antibodies are negative. Peripheral smear shows acanthocytes and burr cells. What is the most likely underlying etiology of this patient's current presentation?
   A. Vitamin deficiency
   B. Alagille syndrome

C. Breast milk jaundice

D. Wilson disease

E. Acute exacerbation of autoimmune hepatitis

2. A 35-year-old woman returns to your office due to 6 months of intermittent upper abdominal pain. She complains of a vague, burning sensation in her upper abdomen that is at its worst after meals. She sometimes also experiences bloating and nausea. Antacids and omeprazole did not relieve her abdominal pain. She has a history of pre-hypertension, which she has been trying to control with diet and exercise. She uses NSAIDs for an occasional headache, but otherwise does not take any medications. Her family is healthy. She does not drink alcohol or smoke cigarettes. She is not married. She was in Mexico about 7 months ago for a work trip. She denies dysphagia, vomiting, weight loss, or change in her stool. Her heart rate is 82 beats/min, respiratory rate is 14/min, and temperature is 99.3°F. Her body mass index is 25 kg/m² and her physical exam is unremarkable other than hemoccult positive stools. What is the next best step in evaluating patient's abdominal pain?

A. Abdominal plain film

B. Abdominal CT scan

C. Consult gastroenterology for endoscopy and/or colonoscopy

D. Stool antigen testing for *H. pylori*

E. No further testing required at this time

ANSWERS: What Would Gunner Jess/Jim Do?

1. WWGJD? A 10-month-old male is brought in by her mother for decreased energy and worsening instability while crawling or walking for the past several weeks. According to the mother, this patient was "yellow" shortly after birth and had dark urine and pale stools. He required a GI procedure at 1 month of age. Since then, the patient has been awaiting a liver transplant. The patient does not take any medications or supplements. On exam, the patient has normal morphologic features, sublingual jaundice, and pale conjunctiva. Laboratory results are notable for hemolytic anemia, hepatobiliary disease, no autoimmune antibodies... BLAH BLAH unconjugated hyperbilirubinemia, decreased haptoglobin, elevated LDH, decreased hemoglobin, elevated ALP, and elevated AST/ALT. Anti-smooth muscle antibody (ASMA), anti-nuclear antibody (ANA), anti-liver kidney microsomal antibodies (anti-LKM), and anti-soluble liver antigen (SLA) antibodies are negative. Peripheral smear shows acanthocytes and burr cells. What is the most likely underlying etiology of this patient's current presentation?

Correct Answer: A

A. This patient is presenting with classic signs and symptoms of hemolytic anemia (fatigue, decreased hemoglobin, unconjugated hyperbilirubinemia, elevated LDH, decreased haptoglobin, jaundice, pale conjunctiva). In this case, the patient has developed hemolytic anemia due to vitamin E deficiency.

This patient had a history of neonatal jaundice as well as a GI procedure. These are classic hints toward biliary atresia, a condition in which bile ducts either fail to form or are destroyed early in life, thereby preventing bile from entering the duodenum. Patients undergo the Kasai procedure within the first few weeks to months of life to restore normal flow of bile and prevent the development of early cirrhosis. However, this procedure frequently eventually fails, and patients may present to clinic or the emergency room with signs and symptoms of fat-soluble vitamin deficiency secondary to a lack of bile in the small bowel, as in this case.

Vitamin E deficiency presents with hemolytic anemia with acanthocytes and Burr cells on peripheral

smear, muscle weakness, and ataxia secondary to spinocerebellar tract and posterior column
degeneration.

B. Alagille syndrome is an inherited disorder characterized by paucity of intrahepatic bile ducts
resulting in cholestatic liver disease, unusual facial
characteristics (saddle nose, wide eyes, etc.),
coloboma, classic butterfly vertebrae, and growth
failure. This patient does not have any of these
characteristics.

C. Although breast milk jaundice is a common cause
of unconjugated hyperbilirubinemia, it does
not cause hemolysis, liver disease, or vitamin
deficiency.

D. Wilson disease may cause hemolytic anemia,
neurologic symptoms such as gait instability, and
liver disease requiring a liver transplant. However, it
does not present at such an early age. Think Wilson
disease in a patient with hepatitis in addition to
neuropsychiatric symptoms and/or renal disease
before the age of 30.

E. Autoimmune hepatitis is characterized by the presence of any of the following antibodies: antismooth
muscle (ASMA), antineutrophil (ANA), antiliver kidney microsomal antibodies (anti-LKM), antisoluble
liver antigen (anti-SLA) antibodies. Autoimmune
hepatitis typically presents later in life with signs
and symptoms of cirrhosis and is much more common in females.

2. WWGJD? A 35-year-old woman returns to your office
due to 6 months of intermittent upper abdominal pain.
She complains of a vague, burning sensation in her
upper abdomen that is at its worst after meals. She
sometimes also experiences bloating and nausea.
Antacids and omeprazole did not relieve her abdominal
pain. She has a history of pre-hypertension which she
has been trying to control with diet and exercise. She
uses NSAIDs for an occasional headache, but otherwise
does not take any medications. Her family is healthy.
She does not drink alcohol or smoke cigarettes. She
is not married. She was in Mexico about 7 months ago
for a work trip. She denies dysphagia, vomiting, weight
loss, or change in her stool. Her HR is 82 beats/min, RR
is 14/min, and temperature is 99.3°F. BMI is 25 kg/m^2.
Physical exam is unremarkable other than hemoccult
positive stools. What is the next best step in evaluating
patient's abdominal pain?

Correct Answer: D

D. This woman presents with a history of chronic, episodic abdominal pain, post-prandial pain, and blood in her stools. This is most consistent with peptic ulcer disease. Since the pain is worse after eating, this is most likely a gastric ulcer (as opposed to a duodenal ulcer, in which pain decreases after eating).

There are many causes of gastric ulcers: long-term NSAID use, smoking, alcohol use, infection (*H. pylori*), increased ICP (Cushing ulcer), and burns (Curling ulcer). It would be important to test this patient for *H. pylori* given her recent history of travel to a low-income area with a high prevalence of infection and persistent symptoms despite appropriate therapy (PPI). Evaluation can be done using urea breath testing and stool antigen testing. Initial therapy includes antibiotics (amoxicillin + clarithromycin) and oral PPI, the combination of which is labeled "triple therapy".

A and B. Imaging is not indicated at this time. Though tumors (i.e., ZES) may be contribute cause ulcers, they are usually in the duodenum or even jejunum and there is low suspicion for this at the time.

C and D. This patient does not have any alarm symptoms (weight loss, dysphagia, persistent vomiting, fatigue, hematochezia) and is under 55 years of age. Thus, there is no need for endoscopy. The patient would, however, need an endoscopy for further evaluation if this does not resolve her symptoms.

Gynecologic Disorders

Hao-Hua Wu, Leo Wang, and Katherine Margo

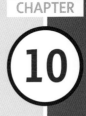
Introduction

Gynecologic disorders may make up as many as 1%–5% of questions on exam day. Prophylactic management of cancer, such as screening tests and when to administer, are common questions you will see on exam day. Make sure also to know the work-up for these screening tests in case something does turn up for "abnormal." For instance, there is a different screening algorithm for patients who have had abnormal cytology on Pap smear than for those who do not.

This chapter is organized into (1) breast disorders, (2) malignant and premalignant neoplasms of the cervix, (3) benign cysts of the vagina and vulva, (4) menstrual and endocrine disorders, and (5) Gunner Practice. Anticipate spending 4–7 hours on this chapter during your first pass, particularly if you have not yet had your ob/gyn rotation.

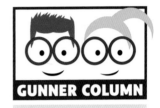

GUNNER COLUMN

Breast Disorders

Infectious, Immunologic, and Inflammatory Disorders

Mastitis

Buzz Words: Focal breast pain + breast erythema + nipple cracking + variations in temperature from one part of breast to another + infectious symptoms (fever, malaise, myalgias)

Clinical Presentation: Presents especially in nursing women as a painful breast ± nipple discharge

PPx: N/A

MoD: Bacteria (most often *Staphylococcus aureus*) enter the breast via small cracks in the skin caused by breast-feeding, causing a superficial infection of breast tissue.

Dx:
1. Physical exam revealing a tender erythematous breast
2. Elevated white blood cell (WBC) count

Tx/Mgmt:
1. Continue to nurse
2. Oral antibiotics. Anti-staphylococcal antibiotics are required. Dicloxacillin or cephalexin is first-line.

Trimethoprim-sulfamethoxazole is indicated if patient is at risk for MRSA

3. If unresponsive to oral antibiotics: intravenous (IV) antibiotics
4. If unresponsive to IV antibiotics: suspect abscess, which requires surgical treatment

Breast Abscess

Buzz Words: Painful palpable fluctuant breast mass + purulent nipple discharge + skin erythema + infectious symptoms (fever, malaise, myalgias)

Clinical Presentation: Presents in breastfeeding females who have had a history of preceding mastitis.

PPx: Can be prevented by timely and appropriate treatment of mastitis and encouraging mother to continue breastfeeding with affected breast.

MoD: Progression of a superficial infection of breast tissue → localized collection of pus and associated tissue destruction.

Dx:

1. Physical exam reveals a warm tender fluctuant breast mass with associated purulent nipple discharge
2. Elevated WBC
3. Ultrasound to localize mass

Tx/Mgmt:

1. Ultrasound-guided needle aspiration of abscess until no collection remains
2. If overlying skin is compromised or if abscess is unresponsive to aspiration: incision and drainage

Benign and Undefined Disorders

Solitary Breast Cyst

Buzz Words: Small rounded or oval fluid-filled sac + nontender + smooth borders

Clinical Presentation: Presents in adult premenopausal and perimenopausal females. Usually asymptomatic and found incidentally. Patients may complain of a breast lump.

PPx: N/A

MoD: Lobule in the terminal ductal lobular unit grows into a fluid-filled mass.

Dx:

1. Ultrasound to visualize mass
2. Aspiration of fluid
3. Mammogram

Tx/Mgmt: Reassurance and observation because most cysts will resolve spontaneously. Drainage of fluid can be performed if the cyst enlarges or becomes painful.

Fibrocystic Change

Buzz Words: Multiple painful bilateral breast masses + straw-colored nipple discharge + fluctuation in size and severity with menstrual cycle

Clinical Presentation: Seen in premenopausal females who have cyclic breast swelling, pain, and tenderness.

PPx: Avoid caffeine (controversial)

MoD: Exaggerated response of breast tissue to physiologic hormonal changes during menstrual cycle.

Dx:

1. History and physical exam
2. Fine-needle aspiration (FNA) of fluid

Tx/Mgmt:

1. OCPs
2. Danazol (androgen agonist), bromocriptine (dopamine agonist), and tamoxifen (selective estrogen antagonist in the breast) may be used in severe cases if OCPs are ineffective
3. Nonsteroidal anti-inflammatory drugs (NSAIDs) for pain

Fibroadenoma

Buzz Words: Firm rubbery nontender round mass + freely moveable + well-circumscribed + often solitary and unilateral + no fluctuation in size with menstrual cycle + slow or no growth (vs. phyllodes tumors which grow rapidly)

Clinical Presentation: Seen in young adult females (late teens and 20s) with no fluctuation in size with menstrual cycle (unlike fibrocystic change).

PPx: N/A

MoD: Benign proliferation of breast epithelium and stroma

Dx:

1. Mammogram to visualize lesion
2. Ultrasound to differentiate solid versus cystic components
3. FNA to confirm Dx

Tx/Mgmt:

1. If asymptomatic: Observation and reassurance because most fibroadenomas will be reabsorbed
2. If mass enlarges or is persistent for more than 3 months: excisional biopsy
3. If mass is very large (>5 cm): FNA to rule out cystosarcoma phyllodes

> **QUICK TIPS**
>
> Fibrocystic change usually fluctuates with the menstrual cycle. Fibroadenomas do not.

Intraductal Papilloma

Buzz Words: Bloody or serosanguinous nipple discharge + no concurrent breast mass

Clinical Presentation: Intraductal papilloma is frequently at the top of the differential whenever bloody nipple discharge is encountered.

PPx: N/A

MoD: Benign growth of epithelial lining (papilloma) arises within the lactiferous ducts (intraductal):

- Papilloma intermittently blocks the duct → non-bloody discharge
- Large papillomas can twist around their stalk → infarction → bloody discharge

Dx:

1. Cytology of discharge to rule out invasive papillary cancer
2. Mammogram to rule out other lesions. Mammogram will not show papilloma due to its small size

Tx/Mgmt: Surgical excision of involved duct

Malignant Neoplasms

Breast Cancer

Buzz Words: Irregular fixed breast mass + spiculated mass on imaging + asymmetric + architectural distortion + retraction of overlying skin and/or nipple + "orange peel" skin texture (peau d'orange) + eczematous lesion of nipple/areola + palpable axillary lymph nodes

Clinical Presentation: This is one of the most high-yield topics of this chapter, particularly for the breast cancer screening guidelines. Patients present with breast lump that is often asymptomatic and found on screening mammography. Patients may have:

- History of ductal carcinoma in situ (DCIS) or lobular carcinoma in situ (LCIS)
- Increased lifetime estrogen exposure due to younger age at menarche, nulliparity, older age of first live birth, older age at menopause, obesity, and long-term (>5 years) use of hormone-replacement therapy
- Prior exposure to ionizing radiation (e.g., treatment of Hodgkin lymphoma during childhood)
- Family history of gynecologic malignancies
- First-degree relatives with breast cancer; risk increases with number of first-degree relatives and early age at time of Dx
- BRCA1/BRCA2 genes are associated with bilateral pre-menopausal breast cancer and ovarian cancer

PPx: US Preventive Services Task Force (USPSTF): Biennial mammograms from age 50 to 74

MoD: N/A

Dx:

1. Screening mammography
2. Needle biopsy or FNA for definitive Dx
3. Staging work-up for metastatic disease

Tx/Mgmt:
1. Lumpectomy
2. Simple mastectomy
3. Radical mastectomy
4. Sentinel lymph node (Table 10.1)

Paget Disease of the Breast

Buzz Words: Eczema (scaling, crusting, ulceration) of the nipple/areolar complex + unilateral + malignant intraepithelial cells (Paget cells) ± concurrent underlying breast cancer (~90% of cases)

Clinical Presentation: Paget disease of the breast typically affects adult females (50s and 60s) with a chief complaint of pain and/or itching of nipple

PPx: N/A

MoD: Malignant cells invade into epidermis of the nipple → inflammation of the nipple → spread to areola → eczematous changes of the nipple/areolar complex

TABLE 10.1 Surgical and Adjuvant Treatment Options for Breast Cancer

	Description	Indications
Lumpectomy	Segmental resection of lesion with margins, leaving most of breast tissue and overlying skin intact	Small breast neoplasms located away from the nipple/areolar complex in a larger breast
Simple mastectomy	Removal of all breast tissue and overlying skin, leaving axillary contents intact	Large breast neoplasms near the nipple/areolar complex in a large breast. Breast neoplasms that occupy most of a small breast
Radical mastectomy	Removal of all breast tissue, overlying skin, axillary contents, and pectoralis minor muscle	Breast neoplasms with lymphatic spread
Sentinel lymph node biopsy	Sentinel lymph node is identified by radioactive tracer injected near the tumor and is then removed and biopsied to assess for metastatic spread of tumor cells	Lumpectomies and simple mastectomies

Dx:

1. Diagnostic biopsy of skin demonstrating the presence of intraepithelial adenocarcinoma cells (Paget cells) within the nipple
2. Mammography to identify an associated mass

Tx/Mgmt: Surgical resection of the lesion

Malignant and Premalignant Neoplasms of the Cervix

Cervical Dysplasia and Management of Abnormal Pap Smears

Definitions:

1. **Cervical dysplasia** = atypical cellular change within the cervical squamous epithelium (seen on cervical cytology or biopsy) due to persistent infection with HPV and active replication of the virus.
2. **Human papillomavirus (HPV)** = a DNA virus with numerous distinct genotypes of differing oncogenic potential and tropism for epithelium of the cervix, vagina, vulva, anus, and oropharynx. HPV is the most common sexually transmitted infection in the United States.
3. **Cervical intraepithelial neoplasia (CIN)** = premalignant dysplasia of cervical squamous epithelium, which encompasses the lower third (CIN 1), lower two-thirds (CIN 2), or greater than two-thirds (CIN 3) of the epithelial thickness. This terminology was used to classify premalignant cervical dysplasia prior to 2012, with the degree of dysplasia (mild, moderate, or severe) increasing from CIN 1 to CIN 3.
4. **Atypical squamous cells of undetermined significance (ASC-US)** = squamous cells seen on cervical cytology specimens ("Pap" smears) that differ from normal epithelial cells but do not meet criteria for a squamous intraepithelial lesion.
5. **Low-grade squamous intraepithelial lesion (LSIL)** = on cervical cytology, squamous cells with mild dysplastic changes such as koilocytosis, nuclear enlargement, and hyperchromasia. On histology (biopsy), a low-grade lesion with mild dysplasia of the lower third of the cervical epithelium (previously CIN 1) or dysplasia of the lower two-thirds of the epithelium (previously CIN 2) that is negative for p16 by immunohistochemistry.
6. **High-grade squamous intraepithelial lesion (HSIL)** = on cervical cytology, squamous cells with moderate-to-severe dysplasia, such as significant nuclear enlargement, size variation, hyperchromasia, and irregularity. On histology, a high-grade lesion

(previously CIN 3) with dysplasia of two-thirds to full thickness of the cervical epithelium, often with markedly dysplastic cells. HSIL also refers to lesions with dysplasia encompassing two-thirds of the epithelium (previously CIN 2) that are positive for p16 by immunohistochemistry.

7. **Atypical squamous cells, cannot exclude high-grade squamous intraepithelial lesion (ASC-H)** = squamous cells seen on cervical cytology that display abnormalities suspicious for HSIL and likely are a mixture of true HSIL and other findings that could mimic HSIL. This cytology finding is associated with a much higher risk of cervical neoplasia than ASC-US.

8. **Atypical glandular cells (AGC)** = endometrial or endocervical glandular cells with dysplastic features that can be seen on cervical cytology and require further investigation either for endometrial or endocervical abnormalities.

9. **"Co-testing"** = simultaneous cervical cytology (Pap smear) examination and high-risk HPV DNA testing performed on the same cervical sample to improve detection of cervical neoplasia. Co-testing is recommended for women after the age of 29.

10. **Reflex HPV testing** = testing for high-risk HPV DNA performed on the same cervical sample used for cytology *only* if results reveal ASC-US. Reflex HPV testing is recommended for women aged 25–29.

Buzz Words: Abnormal Pap smears, history of sexually transmitted infections (STIs), sexually active, acetowhite changes on colposcopy, postcoital spotting

Clinical Presentation:
- Age: 21–65, no testing for HPV or cervical dysplasia recommended prior to 21 or after 65 (if patient has no history of positive Pap smears and is up to date with screening).
- Site of care: Outpatient clinic
- Chief complaint: Asymptomatic
- PMH/PSuH/PFH: N/A
- PSoH: Most risk factors for cervical dysplasia are related to an increased risk of infection with HPV: increased or early onset of sexual intercourse → increased exposure to HPV → increased risk of persistent infection with oncogenic strains of HPV → increased risk of cervical dysplasia and cancer.
  a. Young age at first coitus (early sexual activity)
  b. Multiple sexual partners (risk increases with number of sexual partners)

    c. Sexual intercourse with high-risk partners (partners who have had multiple sexual partners)

    d. History of STIs

    e. History of vulvar or vaginal squamous dysplasia or cancer (also caused by HPV infection)

    f. Early age at first childbirth

    g. Multiparity

    h. Low socioeconomic status

    i. Cigarette smoking (associated with cervical squamous cell carcinoma but not cervical adenocarcinoma)

PPx: HPV vaccination prior to initiation of sexual activity can prevent infection with a select number of HPV strains importantly, many of the oncogenic subtypes such as high-risk HPV genotypes 16 and 18. The recommendations for cervical cancer screening in vaccinated women are the *same* as unvaccinated women.

MoD: Infection of cervical squamous epithelium with HPV → persistence of HPV infection (likelihood of persistence higher in older women, immunosuppressed women, or those infected with high-risk HPV genotypes) → active viral replication causes dysplasia seen on cervical cytology (LSIL) → HPV is eventually cleared or HPV integrates its genome with host DNA causing overexpression of E6/E7 viral oncogenes in cervical epithelium → HSIL → invasive cervical carcinoma.

Dx:

1. **Cervical cytology (Papanicolaou "Pap" smear)** = a screening tool used to assess for premalignant cervical dysplasia or cancer by microscopic evaluation of cytologic features in cells that are scraped off the cervix and endocervical canal during a speculum examination. Newer techniques involve liquid-based preparations rather than the traditional "Pap" smear. The more recent addition of co-testing for high-risk HPV genotypes has improved detection of and risk stratification for cervical cancer

2. **Colposcopy** = a procedure involving a microscope (colposcope) to directly visualize the cervix with higher magnification and take biopsies of any suspicious areas, usually performed when a Pap smear reveals abnormal or undetermined cytology. Cervical biopsies are better able to show squamous epithelial architecture and histology and are more definitive than cytology. During colposcopy, the physician will apply acetic acid to the cervix, which dries out the dysplastic cells more than the normal cells and highlights dysplasia as acetowhite changes

QUICK TIPS

HPV genotypes 16 and 18 are most commonly isolated from HSIL and cervical cancer specimens and are thus designated high-risk (oncogenic) HPV genotypes, in contrast to genotypes 6 and 11, which are most often isolated from anogenital warts or LSIL and are designated low-risk (low oncogenic potential).

Tx/Mgmt of Normal Cytology:
Management is age-dependent:
1. **Women aged 21–24**: Cytology (Pap smear) every 3 years.
2. **Women aged 25–29**: Cytology every 3 years with reflex testing for HP5.
3. **Women aged 30 and above**: Co-testing with HPV is preferred, but cytology every 3 years with reflex testing for HPV is an acceptable alternative.

Tx/Mgmt of Abnormal Cytology: Refer to Gynecologist. The Family Medicine Clinical Subject Exam will not test on specifics of what to do with abnormal Pap smears.

Cervical Cancer

In the United States and other developed countries of the world, cervical cancer has the third highest incidence and mortality rate among gynecologic malignancies, after endometrial and ovarian cancers. However, in developing and underdeveloped nations, cervical cancer has the second highest incidence and mortality rate among *all* malignancies in women, largely due to inadequate vaccination against HPV and insufficient screening for and treatment of early cervical dysplasia. In Africa and Central America, cervical cancer is the number one cause of death by cancer among women.

Cervical cancer can be broken down into two main histological subtypes, squamous cell carcinoma (70%) and adenocarcinoma (25%), with the remainder comprised of less common cervical cancer variants (e.g., adenosquamous, adenoid cystic, undifferentiated). Unlike ovarian and endometrial cancers, which are staged surgically, cervical cancer is staged *clinically* by information obtained from a bimanual pelvic examination and rectal-vaginal examination as well as colposcopy, cystoscopy, proctosigmoidoscopy, X-ray, barium enema, or intravenous pyelogram depending on the patient's clinical presentation. Radioimaging modalities such as computed tomography (CT), transvaginal ultrasound (TVUS), and magnetic resonance imaging (MRI) are not used to stage cervical cancer but can be clinically useful for surgical planning.

Buzz Words: Postcoital spotting + malodorous vaginal discharge + exophytic cervical lesion + history of abnormal Pap smears + lost to follow-up + non-adherence to cervical cancer screening guidelines

Clinical Presentation: Since family medicine emphasizes screening tests more than any other shelf, make sure to learn the cervical cancer screening guidelines well (see above). Patients with cervical cancer can present with postcoital spotting, abnormal vaginal bleeding, malodorous vaginal discharge (due to necrotic tumor), flank tenderness (hydronephrosis caused by tumor invasion into a ureter), constipation (tumor invasion into large bowel).

PPx: HPV vaccination prior to initiation of sexual activity can prevent infection with a select number of HPV strains, importantly many of the oncogenic genotypes such as high-risk HPV genotypes 16 and 18. HPV vaccination is primary prevention against cervical cancer, while screening for cervical dysplasia (Pap smears) is secondary prevention, because removing precursor lesions can prevent development of cervical cancer. Often women who present with cervical cancer in the United States, especially later stages, have been lost to follow-up or were noncompliant with regular cervical cancer screening, and therefore were not treated at earlier stages of cervical dysplasia (LSIL or HSIL).

MoD: ~15 to 25 years from initial infection with HPV to invasive carcinoma

Dx:

1. Cervical biopsy is the best diagnostic procedure and is the appropriate next step if a suspicious cervical lesion is visualized on speculum exam or colposcopy
2. Cervical cytology (Pap smear) is not appropriate for *diagnosing* cervical cancer and can be used only for screening purposes
3. Final diagnosis is confirmed by histologic evaluation of a cervical biopsy
4. Cervical cancer is staged clinically by information obtained from a bimanual pelvic examination and rectal-vaginal examination as well as colposcopy, cystoscopy, proctosigmoidoscopy, X-ray, barium enema, or intravenous pyelogram depending on the patient's clinical presentation
5. Radioimaging modalities such as CT, TVUS, and MRI are not used to stage cervical cancer but can be clinically useful for surgical planning

Tx/Mgmt:

1. Referral to gynecologic oncologist
2. Surgery or radiation

Benign Cysts of the Vagina and Vulva

Bartholin Gland Cyst

Buzz Words: Cystic vulvar mass + 4 o'clock or 8 o'clock position

Clinical Presentation: The bartholin gland cyst is a relatively common vulvar mass that forms due to cystic dilation of an obstructed Bartholin gland duct.

PPx: N/A

MoD: Bartholin glands function to lubricate the vagina and vulva by producing mucus secretions. These ducts open into the vulvar vestibule at 4 and 8 o'clock positions on each side of the vagina and can become obstructed, forming a cyst or an abscess (if infected).

Dx: Clinical diagnosis of finding a soft, painless vulvar mass at the site of a Bartholin gland duct.

Tx/Mgmt:

1. No treatment is required for asymptomatic Bartholin cysts
2. Bartholin cysts that are causing discomfort can be drained (with a high rate of recurrence) or excised for definitive treatment
3. If the cyst is painful, fluctuant, or swollen, it is more likely to be a Bartholin gland abscess, and will require incision and drainage followed by either marsupialization or placement of a catheter to prevent recurrence

Gartner Duct Cyst

Buzz Words: Asymptomatic or incidentally found vaginal mass + anterolateral wall

Clinical Presentation: Gartner duct cyst is a relatively common vaginal mass found along the anterior and lateral vaginal walls that forms due to cystic dilation of an obstructed Gartner duct.

PPx: N/A

MoD: Gartner ducts are remnants of the embryonic mesonephric (Wolffian) ducts that course over the anterolateral aspect of the vaginal canal. Cysts can arise in these ducts if they become obstructed, though they are typically small, asymptomatic, and incidentally found.

Dx:

1. Often an incidental finding on pelvic examination
2. Clinical diagnosis of finding a soft, painless vaginal mass along the anterior or lateral vaginal walls

Tx/Mgmt: Surgical excision is only recommended if the cyst becomes symptomatic.

Menstrual and Endocrine Disorders

Polycystic Ovarian Syndrome (aka Stein-Leventhal Syndrome)

Buzz Words: Hirsutism + acne + male patterned baldness + amenorrhea/oligomenorrhea + multiple cysts in ovaries + acanthosis → polycystic ovarian syndrome (PCOS)

Clinical Presentation: PCOS is a disorder of unknown etiology that is a common cause of secondary amenorrhea. It is diagnosed if patients meet two of three Rotterdam criteria. (1) Laboratory or clinical signs (e.g., male-pattern baldness, acne, or hirsutism) of high serum androgen present. (2) Amenorrhea or oligomenorrhea. (3) Cystic ovaries seen on pelvic ultrasound (string of pearls). Because insulin resistance is a characteristic of PCOS, patients with PCOS are at increased risk of diabetes, dyslipidemia, cardiovascular disease, and metabolic syndrome. In addition, patients have increased risk of endometrial hyperplasia and endometrial cancer.

PPx: (1) None to prevent PCOS, but once patient has PCOS, PPx diabetes and cardiovascular disease.

MoD: Unknown but associated with insulin resistance, cystic ovaries, and hyperandrogenism

Dx:
1. Clinical evaluation (Rotterdam criteria)
2. Pelvic ultrasound of ovaries
3. Testosterone (should be elevated)
4. Follicle-stimulating hormone (FSH)/luteinizing hormone (LH) (should be elevated, LH > FSH so higher LH:FSH ratios)
5. Glucose tolerance test (>140 2-hour GTT → insulin resistance; >200 2-hour GTT → diabetes mellitus)
6. Fasting lipid panel → for all newly diagnosed patients

Tx/Mgmt:
1. Metformin
2. Lifestyle/diet to control diabetes/weight
3. Clomiphene citrate
4. Ketoconazole
5. Spironolactone:
   - Metformin used for PCOS treatment because:
     Prevents T2DM
     Helps lose weight
     Helps induce ovulation in PCOS (mechanism unknown but likely by altering insulin levels to allow for more favorable ovulation)
     Suppresses androgen production by decreasing ovarian gluconeogenesis (helps correct hirsutism)
   - Clomiphene citrate used to induce ovulation; mechanism not elucidated but clomiphene citrate = estrogen analog that improves gonadotropin-releasing hormone (GnRH) and FSH release

Endometriosis

Buzz Words: Chronic pelvic pain (worsens before menses) + dyspareunia + dysmenorrhea for 2 years + regular menses + nodularity over uterosacral area + 27 years old with retroverted uterus + tender adnexa that are normal sized → endometriosis

Thickening of uterosacral ligaments + decreased uterine mobility + infertility + homogenous cystic appearing mass in left ovary → endometriosis

Clinical Presentation: Endometriosis is a condition that results from appearance of endometrial tissue outside the uterus and causes pelvic pain. Ectopic endometrial tissue can implant in a variety of places, including ovaries, appendix, sigmoid colon, round ligament, and broad ligaments. Almost 50% of patients with endometriosis are also infertile.

It is a common cause of secondary dysmenorrhea. Exam will show nodularity of the uterus and tenderness of the adnexa. Pain is from bleeding coming from ectopic endometrium.

PPx: None

MoD: Ectopic endometrial tissue forms on or beneath pelvic mucosal/serosal surfaces → cyclic hyperplasia + degeneration due to response to female sex hormones → chronic hemorrhaging → fibrotic pelvic adhesions → infertility

Dx:
1. Pelvic exam (clinical diagnosis)
2. Beta-human chorionic gonadotropin (hCG)
3. Complete blood count (CBC), BMP
4. TVUS to r/o abnormal anatomy
5. Laparoscopy for definitive diagnosis (will show chocolate-appearing material representing old blood to confirm diagnosis)

Tx/Mgmt:
1. NSAIDs ± combined OCPs
2. If no improvement → laparoscopy to biopsy, ablate or excise implants
3. Progestins, GnRH agonists for those who don't respond to NSAIDs and OCPs
4. Danazol if refractory to laparoscopy
5. Hysterectomy + bilateral salpingoophorectomy (definitve treatment)

Adenomyosis

Buzz Words: Dysmenorrhea + pelvic pain + AUB (menorrhagia) + bulky, globular, tender, boggy uterus + multiparous + >40 year old + symmetrically enlarged → adenomyosis

Clinical Presentation: Adenomyosis is a disorder where there is ectopic glandular tissue found in the myometrium of the uterus. Presents with an enlarged, symmetric uterus and is on the differential for both AUB and dysmenorrhea.

MNEMONIC
The 3 Ds of endometriosis:
dyschezia (pain when defecating) + dysmenorrhea + dyspareunia → endometriosis

QUICK TIPS
Adenomyosis often confused with endometriosis; former occurs >40 years old, latter occurs in <40 years old

PPx: N/A

MoD: Endometrial glands invade uterine musculature → blood deposition between smooth muscle fibers of myometrium → bleeding coming from ectopic endometrium:
- Uterus gradually increases in size 2/2 accumulation of the deposited blood
- Generally does not exceed >12 weeks' gestation size

Dx:
1. Ultrasound
2. Hysterectomy + surgical pathology = definitive diagnosis
3. If >45 years old with irregular menstrual bleeding → endometrial biopsy to r/o malignancy

Tx/Mgmt:
1. NSAIDs
2. OCP or progestin
3. Danazol or continuous GnRH (replicating menopause would lead to decrease in adenomyosis)
4. Endometrial ablation
5. Hysterectomy

Leiomyomata Uteri ("Fibroids," Uterine Leiomyomas)

Buzz Words: Heavy menstrual flow + enlarged, irregular, smooth, freely mobile uterus → fibroids

Enlarged uterus + irregular + mobile uterus with posterior mass + **chronic constipation** + lower abdominal discomfort + >30 years old + **urinary frequency** + difficulty with pregnancy + **heavy, prolonged menstrual bleeding** with normal cycles → leiomyoma aka fibroids

Clinical Presentation: Leiomyomas are the most common pelvic tumors in women, with a higher incidence in black women. They are diagnosed in reproductive-aged women. Symptoms related to uterine leiomyomas generally fade after menopause and leiomyomas shrink as hormone levels decline. The patient's chief complaint is typically heavy and/or prolonged vaginal bleeding, dysmenorrhea, pelvic pain or pressure, or bulk symptoms related to compression of the bladder (urinary frequency) or rectum (constipation). Patients may have a history of infertility or multiple spontaneous abortions (due to submucosal leiomyomas distorting the endometrial cavity), anemia (secondary to severe bleeding).

PPx: Prophylactic treatment of fibroids to prevent future complications is not recommended.

MoD: Proliferation of smooth muscle cells of uterine myometrium

---

QUICK TIPS

Most noteworthy symptom in fibroids is menorrhagia of uterine smooth muscle with various locations in the uterus—submucosal, intramural, subserosal, or cervical.

Dx:
1. Bimanual pelvic exam reveals large, irregularly shaped mobile uterus
2. TVUS → hypoechoic or heterogeneous mass
3. Saline-infused sonohysterography can better characterize intracavitary and submucosal fibroids than TVUS alone
4. MRI, best modality for visualizing multiple leiomyomas in greatly enlarged uteri, is reserved for surgical planning
5. Final diagnosis is confirmed by histologic evaluation of surgical specimen

Tx/Mgmt: There are a variety of treatment modalities for fibroids with the primary goal of eliminating symptoms and improving fertility:
1. Medical management with oral contraceptives or levonorgestrel-releasing intrauterine device (IUD)
2. GnRH agonists
3. Myomectomy
4. Hysterectomy
5. Uterine artery embolization

Mittelschmerz

Buzz Words: Teenager + midcycle unilateral/bilateral lower abdominal pain + normal u/s + normal H&P → mittelschmerz

Clinical Presentation: Mittelschmerz is a phenomenon whereby patients experience pain halfway between their menstrual cycles due to normal follicular enlargement prior to ovulation. As long as the pelvic ultrasound is normal, reassurance is all that is needed for treatment.

PPx: (1) Avoid exposure to unopposed estrogen such as hormone replacement therapy.

MoD: Pain from normal follicular enlargement prior to ovulation

Dx:
1. PE
2. Ultrasound

Tx/Mgmt:
1. Reassurance
2. OCPs if pain is severe enough

Ovarian/Adnexal Torsion

Buzz Words: Acute intermittent abdominal pain + LMP 6 weeks ago with irregular menses + unable to perform pelvic exam due to severe pain + **history of adnexal mass** + impaired ovarian blood flow → torsion of ovarian cyst

Sudden onset pelvic pain (usually R-sided) + unilateral adnexal mass + N/V + low-grade fever → ovarian/adnexal torsion

Sudden onset severe unilateral abdominal pain **following physical activity** + free fluid near ovarian cyst → ruptured ovarian cyst

Clinical Presentation: Ovarian or adnexal torsion is a surgical emergency. This disorder must be ruled out before more benign causes of pelvic pain (e.g., mittelschmerz) can be considered. Patients with masses in the ovary or fallopian tube are more likely to suffer from torsion.

In addition, make sure to rule out ovarian cyst rupture, which occurs in the setting of **physical activity.** Ovarian/adnexal torsion, on the other hand, can occur without physical activity on the shelf.

PPx: Risk factors include (1) pregnancy; (2) ovulation during infertility treatment; and (3) ovarian masses >5 cm.

MoD: Partial or complete torsion of the ovary around the infundibulopelvic (suspensory) ligament of the ovary and the utero-ovarian ligaments:
- More commonly right-sided because left rectosigmoid colon occupies space around the left ovary:
  - **Ovarian torsion** = partial or complete rotation of the ovary around the infundibulopelvic (suspensory ligament of the ovary) and utero-ovarian ligaments
  - **Adnexal torsion** = fallopian tube also twisting along with the ovary

Dx:
1. PE
2. beta-hCG to exclude ectopic pregnancy
3. Ultrasound (shows edematous ovary and **impaired ovarian blood flow**)
4. CBC/BMP

Tx/Mgmt:
1. Laparoscopic surgery for detorsion
2. Salpingo-oophorectomy for obvious adnexal necrosis or suspected ovarian malignancy

Ectopic Pregnancy

Buzz Words: Abdominal pain + amenorrhea + vaginal bleeding + palpable adnexal mass → ectopic pregnancy

Abdominal pain + amenorrhea + vaginal bleeding + orthostatic changes + hypovolemic shock → ruptured ectopic pregnancy

Beta hCG >2000 + **thin endometrial stripe** + "no adnexal masses" + no fetal pole in uterus → ectopic pregnancy

Clinical Presentation: Ectopic pregnancy is a condition in which the fertilized egg matures outside of the uterus (e.g., in the fallopian tube). This is particularly relevant on the Family Medicine shelf because it can present as lower right or left quadrant abdominal pain and be mistaken for a GI disorder. Patients with hypotension or vital signs that suggest hypovolemic shock likely have ruptured ectopic pregnancy, and require admission and surgery. The first test to be ordered is beta-hCG, which would show lower than expected levels. Diagnosis is confirmed with ultrasound. Patients with a history of previous pelvic/tubal surgery, pelvic inflammatory disorder, IUD use, multiple sexual partners, infertility, and in utero DES exposure are more at risk for ectopic pregnancy.

PPx: Avoid risk factors such as (1) previous ectopic/pelvic/tubal surgery; (2) in utero DES exposure; (3) Infertility treatment; (4) IUD use; (5) PID; and (6) multiple sexual partners.

MoD: Ectopic pregnancy is caused by failure of a fertilized egg to implant in the endometrium. Most often occurs in the ampulla of the fallopian tube.

Dx:
1. Pelvic exam
2. Beta-hCG
3. Pelvic ultrasound

Tx/Mgmt:
1. If stable, methotrexate
2. Surgery for hemodynamically unstable patients

GUNNER PRACTICE

1. A 25-year-old woman comes into the physician's office for a well visit. Her asthma is well controlled on albuterol as needed, and she has not had an asthma attack since she was a teenager. She has not played soccer in 1 month since spraining her left ankle, but she is currently able to ambulate without pain to and from work. She denies smoking or drinking alcohol. She is sexually active with one other male partner, and they use condoms for protection. Her last visit 4 years ago showed normal cytology on Pap smear. She has received the HPV vaccine. Her vitals and exam are within normal limits. A screen for HIV and syphilis is

ordered. What is the next best step in management of this patient?

A. Discontinue albuterol
B. Left ankle X-ray to rule out fracture
C. Reassurance, no further work-up needed
D. Pap smear and HPV reflex testing
E. Oral contraceptives

2. A 51-year-old woman comes to the physician complaining of hot flashes that keep her awake at night. She often has to turn the air conditioning on then fall back asleep and is worrying that this is bothering her husband. Patient states that she had her last menstrual period at the age of 49 and has since had difficulty with sexual intercourse. She is worried about her bone health as she has heard that estrogen has a protective effect against fractures. She has not been to the doctors in 2 years, when she received a Pap smear showing no change in cytology. Her vital signs are 120/80, 80 bpm, 98.6 °F and 20 RR. Her physical exam reveals no abnormalities. Her TSH and T3 and T4 are within normal limits. She is interested in trying hormone replacement therapy. In addition to prescribing HRT, what other recommendations should be made for her continued care?

A. Use lubrication for sexual intercourse
B. Use lubrication for sexual intercourse and schedule a mammogram
C. Use lubrication for sexual intercourse, schedule a mammogram, and schedule a colonoscopy
D. Use lubrication for sexual intercourse, schedule a mammogram, schedule a colonoscopy, and schedule a Pap smear
E. Use lubrication for sexual intercourse, schedule a mammogram, schedule a colonoscopy, schedule a Pap smear, and order an MRI to rule out bony pathology

Notes

ANSWERS: What Would Gunner Jess/Jim Do?

1. WWGJD? A 25-year-old woman comes into the physician's office for a well visit. Her asthma is well controlled on albuterol as needed and she has not had an asthma attack since she was a teenager. She has not played soccer in 1 month since spraining her left ankle, but she is currently able to ambulate without pain to and from work. She denies smoking or drinking alcohol. She is sexually active with one other male partner, and they use condoms for protection. Her last visit four years ago showed normal cytology on Pap smear. She has received the HPV vaccine. Her vitals and exam are within normal limits. A screen for HIV and syphilis is ordered. What is the next best step in management of this patient?

   Answer: D. Pap smear and HPV reflex testing.

   Explanation: On the Family Medicine shelf, make sure you know the screening guidelines well for preventable types of cancer, such as cervical cancer. Cervical cancer has the benefit of being slow growing. Thus, screening with a Pap smear for change in cytology only needs to occur once every 3 years from the ages of 21 to 29 (with reflex testing from 25 to 29). Women over the age of 30 require HPV co-testing every 5 years or 3 years with just cytology from the Pap smear. Be on the lookout for these preventative health-type questions anytime there is a female patient who presents to the doctor for a well visit.

   A. Discontinue albuterol → Incorrect. Symptoms were well controlled on current regimen as demonstrated by the lack of asthma attacks in at least 6 years.

   B. Left ankle X-ray to rule out fracture → Incorrect. Patients with sprained ankles that can bear weight (particularly comfortably) don't need an X-ray.

   C. Reassurance, no further work-up needed → Incorrect. Pap smears are indicated at this age to be done every 3 years as long as results are normal.

   E. Oral contraceptives → Incorrect. OCPs can be described as prophylaxis for pregnancy, but are not needed unless requested by the patient.

2. WWGJD? A 51-year-old woman comes to the physician complaining of hot flashes that keep her awake at night. She often has to turn the air conditioning on then

to fall back asleep, and is worrying that this is bothering her husband. The patient states that she had her last menstrual period at the age of 49 and has since had difficulty with sexual intercourse. She is worried about her bone health as she has heard that estrogen has a protective effect against fractures. She has not been to the doctors in 2 years, when she received a Pap smear showing no change in cytology. Her vital signs are 120/80, 80 bpm, 98.6 °F and 20 RR. Her physical exam reveals no abnormalities. Her TSH and T3 and T4 are within normal limits. She is interested in trying hormone replacement therapy. In addition to prescribing HRT, what other recommendations should be made for her continued care?

Answer: C. Use lubrication for sexual intercourse, schedule a mammogram, and schedule a colonoscopy

Explanation: Patients 50 years and older are at higher risk of malignancy and therefore require appropriate recommendations for screening. In this patient, lubrication is recommended for use to prevent pain during sex, something that can happen with vaginal atrophy after menopause. At 50, she is due for a mammogram to screen for breast cancer, something that should be done biennially according to the USPSTF. She is also due for a colonoscopy to rule out colon cancer. She will not need a Pap smear to rule out cervical cancer given a normal test only 2 years ago (should be done once every 3 years or once every 5 years with contesting). While it may be wise to look for bone density to determine risk for osteoporotic fractures, this is done with a DEXA scan and not with MRI.

A. Use lubrication for sexual intercourse → Incorrect. Requires mammogram and colonoscopy as well.

B. Use lubrication for sexual intercourse, schedule a mammogram → Incorrect. Requires colonoscopy as well.

D. Use lubrication for sexual intercourse, schedule a mammogram, schedule a colonoscopy and schedule a Pap smear → Incorrect. Pap smear not indicated since she had had a normal one 2 years ago.

E. Use lubrication for sexual intercourse, schedule a mammogram, schedule a colonoscopy, schedule a Pap smear, and order an MRI to rule out bony pathology. → Incorrect. MRI is not used for prophylactic management.

Notes

Renal, Urinary, and Male Reproductive System

Leo Wang, Jacques Greenberg, Hao-Hua Wu, and Katherine Margo

 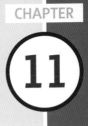

CHAPTER 11

Introduction

Disorders of the renal, urinary, and male reproductive system account for 2%–10% of questions on the Family Medicine exam. These include many common complaints that family physicians encounter, such as hematuria, urinary tract infection, and sexual impotence. As usual, pay attention to the Buzz Words and PPx of each disease mentioned.

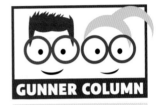

GUNNER COLUMN

A. Chronic Kidney Disease/Chronic Renal Failure

Buzz Words: Renal failure+ diabetes OR HTN OR glomerulonephritis+ glomerular filtration rate (GFR) <15 or patient on dialysis or renal ultrasound (US) → small kidneys

Clinical Presentation:
1. Insidiously increasing blood urea nitrogen and Cr
2. Uremic symptoms:
   a. Nausea/vomiting
   b. Pericarditis
   c. Asterixis
   d. Encephalopathy
   e. Platelet dysfunction:
      i. May manifest as abnormal bleeding
3. Anemia:
   a. Decreased EPO production by poorly functioning kidney

   PMH/PSuH/PFH/PSoH:
   1. Diabetes: most common cause
   2. HTN
   3. Glomerulonephritis

PPx: Fluids, HTN/diabetes control, exercise and diet, smoking cessation

MoD: >3-month insult to the kidneys

Dx:
1. UA
2. BMP
3. Complete blood count
4. US

Tx/Mgmt: Decrease in GFR that accompanies chronic kidney disease (CKD) leads to electrolyte retention and increases incidence of HTN and CHF. Manage these carefully:

1. Manage infections. These are a major cause of mortality in patients with uremia as CKD inhibits humoral and cellular immunity.
2. ACE inhibitors:
   a. First-line
   b. Diuretics may also be necessary
3. EPO when Hgb <10:
   a. Be careful of HTN exacerbations

B. Hematuria

Buzz Words: Blood in urine, blood on dipstick, dipstick positive

Clinical Presentation:

1. Microscopic hematuria:
   a. >3 red blood cell (RBC)/HPF
2. Gross hematuria:
   a. Visible to the naked eye

PPx: N/A

MoD:

1. Microscopic hematuria:
   a. Glomerular disease
2. Gross hematuria:
   a. Postrenal:
      i. Kidney stones
      ii. At beginning of stream:
         1. Urethritis
      iii. At end of stream:
         1. Bladder cancer
         2. Prostatic issues

Dx:

1. Urine dipstick and UA:
   a. Allows for assessment of various causes of hematuria, including renal disease (glomerular or tubular), infection, and non-RBC markers of dipstick positivity (hemoglobin or myoglobin)
2. Cystoscopy, rarely indicated, except as below:
   a. Gross hematuria without evidence of glomerular disease or infection
   b. Microscopic hematuria without evidence of glomerular disease but with high risk of infection
   c. Recurrent urinary tract infections (UTIs)
   d. Obstruction

    e. Irritation without a UTI

    f. Abnormal bladder imaging

Tx/Mgmt: Address underlying cause

Proteinuria

We define proteinuria as urinary excretion of >150 mg protein/day. Nephrotic range proteinuria occurs when urinary excretion exceeds 3.5 g/day. Urinary protein is initially detected by dipstick test. The dipstick is sensitive for albumin. Therefore, it will not detect globulins (e.g., as seen in myeloma).

    Any abnormal dipstick test must be followed up by a urinalysis and 24-hour collection. If the patient is asymptomatic and the proteinuria is transient, then reassurance will suffice. However, if the patient is asymptomatic but the proteinuria is persistent, further testing is required. *Assess blood pressure and examine the urine sediment.* Treat the underlying condition. When a patient becomes symptomatic, the underlying disease must be addressed and ACE inhibitors should be started. *ACE inhibitors minimize the loss of urinary albumin. They should always be started in diabetics with HTN to prevent microalbuminuria.* Patients with proteinuria have weakened immune systems. Therefore, they should be vaccinated against influenza and pneumococcus.

Nephropathies

The Family Medicine shelf will not test you on differences between nephrotic and nephritic syndromes. A basic recognition of the differences between the two is sufficient. In nephrotic syndrome, there is significant protein loss (>3.5 g/day). In nephritic syndrome, there is less protein loss but there is usually hematuria. The manifestations of these diseases are not tested, except in the three cases below. Recognize the following manifestations:

Diabetic Nephropathy

Buzz Words: Kimmelstiel-Wilson nodules + microalbuminuria + LM-mesangial expansion and Kimmelstiel-Wilson nodules in diabetic patient

Clinical Presentation: Nephrotic syndrome in diabetes patients

PPx: Screen for microalbumin with UA upon first diabetes diagnosis, screening should begin within 5 years. Patients should also control **HYPERTENSION**.

   a. Albumin to creatinine ratio from random spot:
      i. >30 mg/g creatinine
   b. 24-hour creatinine clearance:
      i. >30 mg/24 hours
   c. Overnight creatinine collection

MoD: Glomerular hyperfiltration is the earliest renal abnormality seen in diabetes mellitus, but basement membrane thickening is the first to be quantitated.

Dx:
1. UA
2. BMP
3. Biopsy

Tx/Mgmt:
1. Protein restriction
2. Hypertension management:
   a. ACEI/ARB → 130/80
3. Optimize glucose control:
   a. Insulin, HbA1c <6.5%
4. Lower low-density lipoprotein:
   a. <100 mg
5. Aspirin
6. Smoking cessation counseling
7. Anemia management (EPO + iron)

Hypertensive Nephropathy

Buzz Words: Microalbuminuria in hypertensive patient:
   a. benign—thickening of afferent arterioles in patients with long-standing HTN
   b. malignant—rapid decrease in renal fx and increase in blood pressure due to intrarenal injury

Clinical Presentation: Nephrotic syndrome in hypertensive patients; suspect in HTN, African-American, male>female

PPx: Optimal blood pressure (BP) control

MoD: Increased hydrostatic pressure in glomeruli

Dx:
1. UA
2. BMP
3. Biopsy

Tx/Mgmt: Optimal BP control <130/80; BP screening

Renal Stones

Hematuria occurs in over 90% of patients with nephrolithiasis—stones. There are a number of high-yield stone types that you should know and will be reviewed below; but first, let's review some big-picture facts. Urinary stones generally become symptomatic when they lead to urinary tract obstruction. In the acute setting, this may present as colicky flank pain with (or without!) radiation to the groin, hematuria, and nausea and vomiting. However, if the stone develops over a long period of time and leads to urinary tract obstruction chronically, a patient may be asymptomatic. *Obstruction happens at junctions.*

Recall that the ureters cross anteriorly to the iliac vessels at the bifurcation of the common iliac into the internal and external iliac arteries. The *most common and preventable* risk factor for stones is low fluid intake and this is an important point to remember for the Family Medicine shelf. Other risk factors include a family history of stones, predisposing diseases (Crohn's, gout, hyperparathyroidism, RTAs), certain medications, male gender, UTIs with urease-producing bacteria (*Proteus* species), and a *low calcium, high oxalate* diet. As such, someone with kidney stones should drink plenty of fluids (*the most important intervention*), and have low sodium, low protein, and low oxalate in his or her diet. Counterintuitively, he or she should follow a *high calcium* diet.

Diagnosing all stones is done in a similar manner. Urinalysis should be performed. This will allow for the assessment of hematuria, the presence of a UTI or bacteriuria, and the presence of crystals within the urine. A kidney, ureter, and bladder (KUB) radiograph is your first-line in imaging. However, a computed tomography (CT) is more sensitive and is the gold standard in diagnosing a stone. IVPs are only necessary when planning for intervention, and ultrasounds are only used to assess for hydronephrosis or hydroureter, and in pregnant women.

Most stones can be treated with analgesics and fluids. A patient should generally only be referred to an emergency department if his or her pain is noncontrolled on oral analgesics, if anuric (obstruction + solitary kidney = bad news), if there is an accompanying fever, and if the stone is larger than 1 cm. This stone will not pass spontaneously and will thus require intervention. Conversely, stones <0.5 mm generally pass spontaneously.

99 AR

Ureter Anatomy

Calcium Stones

Buzz Words: Radiodense + bipyramidal ovals + biconcave ovals + pain on urination

Clinical Presentation: Most common type of stones, composed of calcium oxalate (most commonly) and calcium phosphate. Suspect in setting of Crohn disease, steatorrhea, sarcoidosis, malignancy, hyperparathyroidism.

PPx: If recurrent, HCTZ; recall that this leads to calcium reabsorption, thus decreasing the amount of calcium in urine

MoD:

1. Hypercalciuria:
   a. Understand that anything that elevates urinary calcium leads to hypercalciuria
2. Hyperoxaluria:
   a. Crohn disease!
      i. Steatorrhea leads to oxalate absorption
   b. B6 deficiency
   c. Drinking too much iced tea!

Dx: See "Renal Stones"

Tx/Mgmt: See "Renal Stones"

Uric Acid Stone

Buzz Words: Radiolucent, flat square plates

Clinical Presentation: Suspect in gout, tumor lysis syndrome

PPx: Allopurinol

MoD: Low urine pH allows formation

Dx: See "Renal Stones"

Tx/Mgmt: See "Renal Stones"; also, add potassium citrate to alkalinize the urine

A. Struvite Stones

Buzz Words: Radiodense, staghorn calculi + rectangular prisms

Clinical Presentation: See above, happens in UTIs with urease-producing organisms, most commonly *Proteus*

PPx: Suppressive antibiotics

MoD: Urease organisms split urea into ammonia → alkaline urine

Dx: See "Renal Stones"

Tx/Mgmt: See "Renal Stones"; be careful for a patient with a fever, as this may be an indication for hospitalization.

B. Cystine Stones

Buzz Words: Radiolucent "stop sign" stones

Clinical Presentation: Least common type of stone seen in cystinuria

PPx: Acetazolamide

MoD: Defective amino acid transport at brush border

Dx: See "Renal Stones":
   a. FU with urinary sodium nitroprusside test

Tx/Mgmt: Recurrence is common

Vascular Pathology Affecting the Upper Urinary Tract

Renal Artery Stenosis

Buzz Words: Sudden onset HTN + HTN nonresponsive to medical therapy + malignant hypertension, "string of beads"

Clinical Presentation: Refractory hypertension in young patient (woman):
  a. MCC of secondary HTN

PPx: NA

MoD: Decreased renal blood flow to the juxtaglomerular apparatus leads to activation of the renin-angiotensin-aldosterone system:
  a. In a young woman, think **fibromuscular dysplasia** ← high yield for the Family Medicine shelf:
    i. "String of beads"
    ii. Non-inflammatory, non-atherosclerotic
    iii. May involve the carotid artery and lead to ischemic brain symptoms
  b. Elderly man w/ numerous cardiac/peripheral artery problems → **atherosclerosis**

Dx:
1. Renal arteriogram gold standard:
   a. Do not use in patients with renal insufficiency
2. Duplex US:
   a. May indicate elevated flow velocities. Good initial test
3. Magnetic resonance angiogram:
   a. Use for patients with renal insufficiency

Tx/Mgmt:
1. Percutaneous transluminal angioplasty is initial treatment
2. Various trials have failed to show benefit for renal artery stenting
3. Surgical bypass may be necessary if angioplasty fails

Infectious Disorders of the Upper Urinary Tract

Pyelonephritis

Buzz Words: White blood cell (WBC) casts + costovertebral angle tenderness + vesicoureteral reflux (VUR)

Clinical Presentation: Dysuria, ± hematuria, frequency/urgency, suprapubic tenderness (all symptoms of cystitis, may or may not be present), fevers/chills, flank pain, CVA tenderness. Suspect in diabetes, females (shorter urethra), sexual intercourse, Foley catheter, VUR

PPx: A vesicoureterogram is indicated to rule out VUR in all males with a UTI to prevent chronic pyelonephritis. If VUR is found, treat low grade with long-term abx until child "grows out" of it or with surgical reimplantation if high grade.

MoD: *Escherichia coli* is most common, but other gram-negative bugs including *Proteus, Klebsiella, Enterobacter*, and *Pseudomonas*, especially in those patients with Foley catheters or those living in nursing homes.

Dx: Ua/UCx on all patients with suspected pyelonephritis. Look for evidence of pyuria (WBC in urine), bacteriuria, and WBC casts:

a. Perform imaging studies if treatment fails after 48–72 hours or in *any* patient with complicated pyelonephritis, a history of nephrolithiasis, or unusual findings.

Tx/Mgmt:

1. Uncomplicated: Bactrim or cipro:
   a. OK for outpatient
2. Complicated (very ill, elderly, pregnant, unable to tolerate PO meds, significant comorbidities, or if uroseptic): admit + IV amp/gent or cipro
3. Recurrent with same organism: treat for 6 weeks

Cystitis (Lower Urinary Tract Infection)

Buzz Words: Honeymoon + catheter + dysuria (burning on urination) + frequency, urgency + suprapubic tenderness + occasional fever

Clinical Presentation: Women>> men; Suspect in: pregnancy—always treat! In-dwelling catheters, diabetes—increases the risk of ascension to kidneys, structural abnormality

PPx: Bladder infection

MoD: Usually ascending infection from the urethra:

a. *E. coli*—most common cause
b. *S. saprophyticus*—sexually active young woman
c. *Enterococcus, Klebsielle, Proteus, Pseudomonas, Enterobacter*—catheter

Dx:

1. Urine dipstick
2. Leukocyte esterase—indicates white blood cells in urine (pyuria)
3. Nitrite—positive for Gram-negative bacteria. *Negative nitrite does not exclude cystitis.*

Tx/Mgmt:

1. Asymptomatic—two successive positive cultures with >10^5 CFUs:
   a. Treated only if patient is pregnant or going to have urologic surgery

2. Uncomplicated:
    a. Empiric treatment is appropriate
    b. Oral trimethoprim/sulfamethoxazole (TMP/SMX) is first-line
    c. Nitrofurantoin or fosfomycin or fluoroquinolones
3. Complicated—structural abnormalities or any of the following:
    a. Male sex:
        i. Same treatment as uncomplicated cystitis, but treat for longer
        ii. Consider further workups
    b. Diabetes, renal failure
    c. Pregnancy:
        i. Avoid fluoroquinoles
        ii. Increase duration of treatment
    d. Pyelonephritis within the past year
    e. Obstruction
    f. In-dwelling catheter, stent, or nephrostomy tube
    g. Antibiotic-resistant organism
    h. Immunocompromise
    i. Recurrent:
        i. TMP/SMX after sex or low dose for 6 months

Infectious

Urinary Tract Infection (Cystitis/Pyelonephritis)

Buzz Words: Fever + pain during urination + cloudy/foul-smelling urine + frequent urination or wetting bed + vomiting

Clinical Presentation: UTIs are a common problem in young children, with girls getting them more commonly than boys (10:1). Most are not serious, but can lead to kidney infections and damage. Many UTIs are caused by vesicoureteral reflux. Uncircumcised boys are also at greater risk of UTIs. Infection may be limited to bladder (**cystitis**) or kidney (**pyelonephritis**). UTIs in infants can be the first sign of an obstructive anomaly or severe vesicoureteral reflux.

PPx: Circumcision in boys

MoD: Ascent from fecal flora in older children, younger children can get UTIs from bacteremia

Dx:

1. UA
2. UCx
3. Urine ultrasound for all children <24 months
4. VCUG/radionuclide cystography in non-responders to antibiotics
5. Dimercaptosuccinic acid scan of kidney

Tx/Mgmt: Cystitis:

1. Amoxicillin
2. TMP/SMX

Pyelonephritis:

1. Cefixime/cefotaxime
2. Ampicillin + Gentamicin

Urethritis

Buzz Words: Painful urination in children

Clinical Presentation: While urethritis is another type of urinary tract infection, it is specifically localized to the urethra and is typically caused by either gonorrhea (gonococcal urethritis) or *Chlamydia* (chlamydial urethritis). Other

TABLE 11.1 Outpatient Management of Pediatric Urinary Tract Infections (Oral Therapy)*

Common Pathogens	Type of Infection	Drug	Dosage	Min Length of Therapy (Days)
Escherichia coli; Enterobacter, Klebsiella, Proteus sp; group B streptococcus (neonates)	Cystitis	Amoxicillin	<3 months: 20–30 mg/kg per day bid ≥3 months: 25–50 mg/kg per day bid Adolescents: 250 mg tid or 500 mg bid	3–7
		Amoxicillin-clavulanate[†]	<3 months: 30 mg/kg per day bid ≥3 months: 25–45 mg/kg per day bid Adolescents: 875/125 mg bid	
		Cefixime	16 mg/kg per day bid × 1 day then 8 mg/kg per day bid thereafter	
		Cephalexin	25–50 mg/kg per day qid (max: 4 g)	
		TMP/SMX[‡]	≥2 months: 8–10 mg/kg per day bid Adolescents: 160 mg bid	
	Acute pyelonephritis	Recommended therapy for cystitis	See above OR	10
		Ciprofloxacin	Infants > 1 year: 20–30 mg/kg per day bid (max: 1.5 g/day)	

*All dosages are suggestions only. Some antibiotics will require adjustment in the presence of renal impairment. For pregnant adolescents, clinicians should review pregnancy risk factors prior to administration. All patients should be screened for drug allergies.

[†]Amoxicillin-clavulanate dose is based on the amoxicillin component.

[‡]TMP/SMX dose is based on the trimethoprim component. Not recommended for patients ≤2 months or patients who have renal insufficiency. Empiric use of TMP/SMX is not recommended if regional resistance to *E. coli* is ≥20%.

max: Maximum; *min*: minimum; *sp*, species; *TMP-SMX*, trimethoprim/sulfamethoxazole; *UTI*, urinary tract infection.

causes are less important for the Pediatric shelf, but include *E. coli*, adenoviruses, CMV, HSV, GBS, MRSA, or *Trichomonas*.

PPx: Proper perineal hygiene

MoD: Perianal spread

Dx:

1. UA
2. UCx

Tx/Mgmt: Antibiotic treatment for gonorrhea (ceftriaxone) or chlamydia (azithromycin, doxycycline).

QUICK TIPS

Some children will present with idiopathic urethritis. It is thought to be an autoimmune phenomenon and can be treated with steroids

Interstitial Cystitis (Painful Bladder Syndrome)

Buzz Words: Urinary frequency/urgency + abdominal/pelvic pain associated with **specific food/drinks**

Clinical Presentation: Disease is co-morbid with diseases like fibromyalgia, allergic and gastrointestinal problems (irritable bowel syndrome), and vulvodynia in women. Can also be caused by vesicoureteral reflux, so presence in a young child may raise suspicion for anatomic abnormality or obstruction. Interstitial cystitis is often misdiagnosed as bacterial cystitis.

PPx: N/A

MoD: Unknown, but thought to be related to autoimmunity or neurologic damage. Others think it is caused by toxin production in urine that inhibits bladder epithelial proliferation.

Dx: Typically a diagnosis of exclusion.

1. UA
2. UCx
3. US
4. Voiding diaries
5. Cystoscopy and hydrodistension

Tx/Mgmt:

1. Conservative/dietary management:
   a. that is, cranberry juice
2. Calcium glycerophosphate
3. Amitryptyline
4. Hydroxyzine/cimetidine
5. Surgical intervention (diversion, augmentation, cystectomy)

Epididymitis

Buzz Words: Testicular torsion + fever, pyuria + tender spermatic cord + pain with urination + pain/swelling in testicles, sexually transmitted in boys >14 year old

Clinical Presentation: While epididymitis does not threaten the testicle, testicular torsion must be ruled out emergently. Therefore, one must obtain a diagnostic US immediately. Once torsion has been excluded, diagnostic tests for epididymitis may be run.

PPx: N/A

MoD: *E. coli* infection from perianal spread or sexually transmitted infection (STI) from gonorrhea/*Chlamydia*

Dx:
1. Physical exam
2. US

Tx/Mgmt: Antibiotic treatment (ceftriaxone/azithromycin/doxycycline for gonorrhea/chlamydia urethritis)

Prostatitis

Buzz Words: Low back pain + recent UTI + frequent urination

Clinical Presentation: *Prostatitis can occur* secondary to STIs or from coliform bacteria. In a young child the most common pathogen is *E. coli* but in an older boy >14, the most common cause is STI. On digital rectal exam, one will feel a "boggy, tender prostate" and UA/UCx will be abnormal. Treatment can be with bactrim or ciprofloxacin. Acute prostatitis *may* lead to slight elevations in prostate-specific antigen (PSA), so do not be fooled into thinking a patient has prostate cancer if he does not fit the clinical picture. Chronic prostatitis may be asymptomatic, and diagnosis is made when WBCs are found in prostatic secretions. Chronic prostatitis must be treated with long-term ciprofloxacin or another fluoroquinolone.

PPx: Barrier contraception

MoD: Perianal or sexual transmission

Dx:
1. UA/UCx
2. DRE
3. Cystoscopy
4. Semen culture
5. US

Tx/Mgmt:
1. Antibiotic treatment (bactrim, ciprofloxacin, though varies by acute vs. chronic and etiology).
2. Chronic prostatitis → ciprofloxacin/fluoroquinolone.

Neoplasms

Prostate Cancer

Buzz Words: Urinary obstruction + bony metastasis

Clinical Presentation: Second most common cancer in men; risk factors-age (#1), African-American, high-fat diet, family history, exposure to herbicides and pesticides
a. Early—asymptomatic. No urinary obstruction because of peripheral location of tumor:
    i. Treat with 5-alpha reductase inhibitor, such as finasteride
        1. Decreases libido and may lead to erectile dysfunction
    ii. May also use alpha blockers such as prazosin:
        1. May lead to orthostatic hypotension
b. Late—urinary obstruction
c. Very late—urinary obstruction + bone metastasis:
    i. Vertebral bodies #1
    ii. Pelvis
        1. Long bones

PPx: (1) 2012 USPSTF guideline recommends against PSA, although PSA could be discussed on an individualized basis (e.g., risk of false positive, leading to unnecessary invasive biopsy). (2) Discuss prostate cancer screening at age 50 for all men. If a man has had a first-degree relative with prostate cancer, start at age 45. If they have had more than one first-degree relative with prostate cancer, start at 40. (3) DRE annually after age 50. (4) Abnormal → transrectal ultrasound (TRUS).

MoD: Adenocarcinomas (90%) develop in the periphery and move centrally

Dx: TRUS + bone scan, plain radiographs of pelvis and spine, CT pelvis

Tx/Mgmt:
1. Localized:
    a. Watchful waiting
    b. Prostatectomy:
        i. Complications include erectile dysfunction and urinary incontinence
2. Locally invasive:
    a. Radiation therapy:
        i. Radiation therapy also beneficial in managing bone pain in patients undergoing orchiectomy
    b. Antiandrogens:
        i. Flutamide
3. Metastatic:
    a. Reduce testosterone in body:
        i. Orchiectomy
        ii. Antiandrogens:

QUICK TIPS

Benign prostatic hyperplasia occurs due to central proliferation of the prostate and thus leads to urinary obstruction.

99 AR

USPSTF guidelines may soon change with regards to PSA

1. Flutamide
iii. Luteinizing hormone-releasing hormone agonists:
1. Leuprolide
iv. Gonadotropin-releasing hormone antagonist:
1. Abarelix, cetrorelix

Sexual Dysfunction

Sexual dysfunction is a common complaint on the Family Medicine shelf, and you will most likely get one or two questions. There are many types of sexual dysfunction, which include those due to impotence, premature ejaculation, dyspareunia (pain), and arousal disorders. The most important on the Family Medicine shelf is erectile dysfunction. Always ensure that the cause is not psychological, and always begin with sildenafil.

Impotence/Erectile Dysfunction

Buzz Words: *Persistent* inability to maintain erection
Clinical Presentation: Upper-middle-aged men, suspect in diabetes, dyslipidemia, atherosclerotic disease, anxiety
PPx: Diabetic and lipid control
MoD: If organic, then a vascular pathology is usually at play. The same atherosclerotic process that leads to peripheral vascular disease also affects the hypogastric artery.
Dx: Clinical
Tx/Mgmt:
1. Psychological (male factor)—couples therapy
2. Organic—PDE5 inhibitors (sildenafil)

A. Premature Ejaculation
Buzz Words: Persistent ejaculation prior to or immediately upon penetration
Clinical Presentation: Men at any age, anxiety
PPx: NA
MoD: Usually secondary to anxiety
Dx: Clinical
Tx/Mgmt:
1. Selective serotonin reuptake inhibitors
2. Psychotherapy

B. Dyspareunia
Buzz Words: Pain on intercourse
PPx: NA

MoD: Psychological. Be on the lookout for past trauma or abuse.

Dx: Rule out all medical causes of pain

Tx/Mgmt: Psychotherapy

C. Arousal disorder

Buzz Words: Absence of three of the following for 6 months *leading to distress*:
   a. Interest in sexual activity
   b. Sexual/erotic thoughts
   c. Initiation/reception of sexual activity
   d. Excitement and pleasure with sexual activity
   e. Sexual arousal in response to both internal and external stimuli
   f. Genital and nongenital sensations

PPx: NA

MoD: Psychological

Dx: Clinical

Tx/Mgmt:
1. Flibanserin
2. Psychotherapy

99 AR

Article about flibanserin

GUNNER PRACTICE

1. A 51-year-old man presents to your office for an annual wellness exam. He asks you about recommendations about prostate cancer screening as one of his friends recently died of prostate cancer. He has never had a family member with prostate cancer. Which of the following is the most appropriate prostate screening in this man?
   A. All men should have digital rectal exams after the age of 50.
   B. All men should have PSA screening after the age of 50.
   C. All men should have digital rectal exams after the age of 50 only if they have had a first-degree relative with prostate cancer.
   D. All men should have PSA screening after the age of 50 only if they have had a first-degree relative with prostate cancer.
   E. Prostate screening is not indicated.

2. A 26-year-old man comes to your office asking for Viagra. He says that he is unable to sustain erections when he has sex with his girlfriend due to "anxiety from school." You note that he has a recurrent history of panic attacks and was previously diagnosed with generalized

anxiety disorder. Which of the following should you say to this patient?

A. "How many times a week do you have sex?"
B. "Do you wear protection?"
C. "Do you get erections at night?"
D. "You have nothing to worry about, this is natural."
E. "Tell me more about your performance in school."

Notes

ANSWERS: What Would Gunner Jess/Jim Do?

1. WWGJD? A 51-year-old man presents to your office for an annual wellness exam. He asks you about recommendations about prostate cancer screening as one of his friends recently died of prostate cancer. He has never had a family member with prostate cancer. Which of the following is the most appropriate prostate screening in this man?

Answer: A. All men should have digital rectal exams after the age of 50. Discuss prostate cancer screening at age 50 for all men. If a man has had a first-degree relative with prostate cancer, start at age 45. If they have had more than one first-degree relative with prostate cancer, start at 40. DRE is recommended annually after age 50.

    B. All men should have PSA screening after the age of 50 → Incorrect. PSA screening is no longer recommended.

    C. All men should have digital rectal exams after the age of 50 only if they have had a first-degree relative with prostate cancer → All men should be receiving a DRE after the age of 50 with or without a first-degree relative with prostate cancer.

    D. All men should have PSA screening after the age of 50 only if they have had a first-degree relative with prostate cancer → PSA screening is recommended for patients with a first-degree relative with prostate cancer but this is not applicable to this patient.

    E. Prostate screening is not indicated → Prostate screening from DRE is indicated for patients over the age of 50.

2. WWGJD? A 26-year-old man comes to your office asking for Viagra. He says that he is unable to sustain erections when he has sex with his girlfriend due to "anxiety from school." You note that he has a recurrent history of panic attacks and was previously diagnosed with generalized anxiety disorder. Which of the following should you say to this patient?

Answer: C. "Do you get erections at night?" This is the most important question you can ask for erectile dysfunction (ED). Most ED is psychologic and not physiologic, especially in patients with co-morbid psychiatric disorders, like anxiety. Patients like this one would not benefit from Viagra, which would enhance blood flow in patients who have physiologic ED from impairment in blood flow.

A. "How many times a week do you have sex?" → This is unnecessary and invasive, although important to understand from a social history context.
B. "Do you wear protection?" → This is a conversation to have later, but warning about barrier contraception is a generally good practice to have.
D. "You have nothing to worry about, this is natural." → No, this is not natural. He is 26.
E. "Tell me more about your performance in school." → While his anxiety in school warrants further follow-up, the topic at hand to be discussed should pertain to his ED.

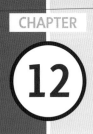

Disorders of Pregnancy, Childbirth, and the Puerperium

Hao-Hua Wu, Leo Wang, and Katherine Margo

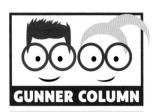

Introduction

For the Family Medicine shelf, disorders of pregnancy, childbirth, and puerperium comprise 1%–5% of questions. Specifically, expect to be tested on concepts related to prenatal care (e.g., including screening for diabetes), high-yield immunizations and screening tests needed, and medication during pregnancy. Background information that would be useful to know is the concept of gestational age and the definition of preterm labor (any labor that occurs <37 weeks gestation). It is also important to remember that preterm labor (which can be seen when there is fluid in the vaginal canal that turns the nitrazine paper blue) is a risk factor for myriad complications, including developmental delay and respiratory distress syndrome.

Prenatal Care

Nutrition During Pregnancy

Buzz Words: Folate supplementation + iron supplementation + weight gain → three key nutritional factors during pregnancy

Clinical Presentation: There is an increasing number of women of reproductive age who have a burden of maternal and fetal complications during pregnancy due to problems such as malnutrition or obesity. For instance, being underweight contributes to increased risk of pre-term birth, low-birth weight, and maternal death. Forgetting to consume enough folate during pregnancy can lead to a neural tube defect. On the shelf, you are expected to know the general outline on how to counsel mom during pregnancy in terms of nutrition.

PPx: (1) Folate supplementation. (2) Iron supplementation (sometimes within multivitamin pill). (3) Increased dietary intake of carbohydrates and proteins. (4) Avoid alcohol and cigarette smoke.

MoD: N/A

Dx:

1. Assess ABCDs of nutrition:
   - Anthropometric factors (weight, height, etc.)

- Biochemical factors (anemia) via complete blood count and basic metabolic panel
- Clinical factors (lifestyle)
- Dietary risks
2. Always assess the woman's understanding of pregnancy and expectations.

Tx/Mgmt: Dietary and lifestyle modifications for patients who are too obese or malnourished.

Immunizations and Screenings

Ideally all pregnant women should already be immunized against **hepatitis B**, influenza, **rubella**, pertussis, and varicella. During pregnancy, patients should receive Tdap and influenza vaccines. Tdap is recommend based on history of immunization. Tdap immunized patients are given Tdap at 27-36 weeks gestation. Patients with questionable immunization status are given 3 doses: first dose at 20 weeks gestation, second dose one month after the first, and third dose six-twelve months after the first. Rubella and varicella vaccines cannot be given during pregnancy since they are live-virus vaccines. Two of the most important things to screen for are gestational diabetes and Rh compatibility. Aneuploidy with quad testing is also often tested for.

Gestational Diabetes

Buzz Words: Gestational diabetes + polyhydramnios + preeclampsia + spontaneous abortion → maternal complications of gestational diabetes

Shoulder dystocia 2/2 macrosomia + hypocalcemia + hypoglycemia + polycythemia + NTD + hyperbilirubinemia + enlarged organs → fetal complications of gestational diabetes

Clinical Presentation: Gestational diabetes is elevated blood sugar during pregnancy. It is unknown why it occurs but is thought to be 2/2 to insulin resistance arising from human placental lactogen (hPL), estrogen, and progesterone. For prenatal care, it is routine to screen for gestational diabetes with an oral glucose tolerance test. Control of blood sugar is important to minimize the maternal complications (e.g., polyhydramnios + spontaneous abortion + preeclampsia) and fetal complications (e.g., macrosomia + hypoglycemia + polycythemia + neural tube defects) that may occur. On the shelf, make sure to know the complications well (included in the Buzz Words).

An important concept to consider is that maternal hyperglycemia can affect the fetus differently depending on the trimester. If mom has gestational diabetes during the first trimester, she is at risk for spontaneous abortion while the fetus is at risk for small left colon syndrome (inability to pass meconium), neural tube defects, and congenital heart disease.

If mom has gestational diabetes during the second and third trimester, the fetus develops hyperinsulinemia leading to four main complications:
1. Macrosomia (big head), which can lead to traumatic birth injuries like shoulder dystocia, Erb palsy, and brachial plexus injury
2. Big organs (e.g., cardiomegaly)
3. Polycythemia 2/2 more red blood cell mass to supply the enlarged organs
4. Hypoglycemia as a neonate

QUICK TIPS
Newborns of patient with gestational diabetes have **hypo**glycemia because of the **hyper**insulinemia compensating for mom's high blood sugar. Once newborn is no longer attached by umbilical cord, the insulin to blood sugar ratio becomes too high.

PPx: (1) **OGTT screening test** (50 g load + measurement at 1 hour, if >130 mg/dL, second 3 hour 100 g GTT administered). (2) Nonstress tests, biophysical profiles, and kick counts after 32 weeks. (3) Postpartum screening and insulin.

MoD: Unknown but associated with insulin resistance that can arise from the influence of hPL, estrogen and progesterone

Dx:
1. OGTT
2. Plasma glucose (two fasting readings >126 mg/dL)
3. A1c for existing diabetics

Tx/Mgmt:
1. Blood glucose daily monitoring
2. Insulin
3. Glyburide
4. If polycystic ovary syndrome (PCOS), give metformin
5. Induce if >39 weeks, v1. C-section if severe macrosomia

Rh Isoimmunization for Incompatibility

Buzz Words: Rh- mother + Rh+ fetus → Rh incompatibility
Mom's second pregnancy + neonatal unconjugated hyperbilirubinemia + neonatal anemia + neonatal positive Coombs test → erythroblastosis fetalis

Clinical Presentation: Rh incompatibility refers to the phenomenon whereby an Rh- mother develops antibodies to Rh factor from carrying an Rh+ fetus. While this **does not affect the first pregnancy** with such a mismatch, the second pregnancy with an Rh+ fetus is at risk for erythroblastosis fetalis, hemolytic anemia of the fetus 2/2 attack from maternal red blood cell

GG AR
Rh factor basic science review video

FOR THE WARDS
Anti-D immunoglobulin is called RhoGAM on the wards

(RBC) antibodies. Prophylactic measures, known as Rh isoimmunization, will likely be 1 or 2 questions on the shelf. Make sure to know the indications for anti-D immunoglobulin administration to an unsensitized Rh- mother, which include:

1. First dose at 28 weeks gestation
2. Second dose within 72 hours of delivering Rh+ infant (e.g., live birth, stillborn, spontaneous abortion)
3. Ectopic pregnancy
4. Vaginal bleeding in the second and third trimester

PPx: (1) If woman is Rh-, anti-D immunoglobulin adminis- tration at 28 weeks pregnancy and within 72 hours of delivery, stillborn or spontaneous abortion.

MoD: Rh- mother and Rh+ father make Rh+ fetus → moth- er's immune system develops antibodies to Rh factor → Rh+ antibodies attack fetal red blood cells → erythro- blastosis fetalis:

- The mechanism for why the anti-D immunoglobulin helps prevent erythroblastosis fetalis is not well understood

Dx:

1. RhD antigen test for fetus and mom to determine Rh+ or Rh-
2. Kleihauer-Betke test to know how much anti-D immu- noglobulin is needed postpartum
3. Ultrasound of middle cerebral artery peak systolic velocity to monitor fetal anemia

Tx/Mgmt:

1. Counseling
2. Treatment of maternal diabetes

Aneuploidy Disorders

Aneuploidy disorders are disorders caused by an abnor- mal number of chromosomes. These are high-yield on the Family Medicine shelf because they are part of the prophy- lactic management of expectant mothers at 15–20 weeks gestation with what is known as the quad screen, a test that measures four variables Table 12.1:

1. Alpha fetal protein (AFP, increased in neural tube defects, decreased in trisomy 21 and 18)
2. Estriol
3. hCG
4. Inhibin A

    Depending on the levels of these four measurements, one can ascertain one of four aneuploidy disorders: Down syndrome (trisomy 21), Edward syndrome

FOR THE WARDS
Anti-D given at Twen-D-eight weeks

FOR THE WARDS
Erythroblastosis fetalis = hemo- lytic anemia of the neonate 2/2 maternal RBC antibodies

99 AR
Summary of quad screen

99 AR
How to read quad screen

TABLE 12.1 Quad Screen Results

Quad screen results	AFP	hCG	Inhibin A	Estriol
Down syndrome	Decreased	Increased	Increased	Decreased
Edward syndrome	Decreased	Decreased	Normal	Decreased
Turner syndrome	Decreased	Decreased (increased with hydrops fetalis)	Decreased	Decreased (increased with hydrops fetalis)

AFP, Alpha fetal protein.

(trisomy 18) Patau syndrome (trisomy 13), and Turner syndrome (XO).

Down Syndrome

Buzz Words: Newborn + sandal-gap toes + hypotonia + flattened nasal bridge + small, rotated cup-shaped ears + small size + **simian creases** + epicanthic folds + oblique palpebral fissures → Down syndrome

Clinical Presentation: Down syndrome (aka trisomy 21) is the constellation of signs and symptoms that occur 2/2 presence of three copies of chromosome 21. The most high-yield Buzz Words are sandal-gap toes and simian crease of the hands. This is very frequently tested on the shelf exam and is seen in Ob/Gyn, Medicine, Surgery, Neurology, and Psychiatry. For the Pediatrics shelf, just be able to identify the newborn Buzz Words. You may also be tested on the medical complications of Down syndrome that affect the pediatric population, such as increased risk of ALL, atlantoaxial instability, as well as cardiac and gastrointestinal (GI) signs that can present at birth:

1. Ventricular septal defect (e.g., "holosystolic murmur")
2. Atrial septal defects (e.g., "fixed split S2" and "low-grade diastolic murmur")
3. Endocardial defects
4. Hirschprung disease (e.g., "failure to pass meconium")
5. Intestinal atresia
6. Annular pancreas
7. Imperforate anus

PPx: More likely tested on Ob/Gyn instead of Pediatrics shelf, but good to know for the wards. (1) First trimester: Pregnancy-associated plasma protein A (PAPP-A) and free beta hCG (known as the combined test) = screening against Down syndrome; positive if high hCG and low PAPP-A. (2) First trimester: Nuchal translucency and presence/absence of nasal bone on ultrasound = screening against Down syndrome. (3) Second semester: quad screening test. (4) Avoid pregnancy during advanced maternal age.

MoD: Non-disjunction of chromosome 21 → trisomy 21

Dx:
1. Karyotype analysis with amniocentesis if quad screening shows decreased AFP/estriol and increased hCG and inhibin A
2. Echo for cardiac defects
3. Abdominal ultrasound for abdominal defects

Tx/Mgmt:
1. Supportive
2. Surgery to repair cardiac or abdominal defects

Edward Syndrome (Trisomy 18)

Buzz Words: Rocker bottom feet + VSD + overlapping flexed fingers + horseshoe kidney → trisomy 18

Clinical Presentation: Trisomy 18 is aneuploidy of chromosome 18 that causes rocker bottom feet, horseshoe kidney, and VSD.

PPx: (1) Quad screen test

MoD: Non-disjunction of chromosome 18

Dx: If quad screen positive, karyotype with amniocentesis

Tx/Mgmt: Surgery for VSD

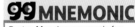

Patau Syndrome (Trisomy 13)

Buzz Words: Newborn + cleft lip + polydactyly → Patau syndrome

Clinical Presentation: Trisomy 13 is aneuploidy of chromosome 13 that causes cleft lip and polydactyly of the newborn. Signs and symptoms can be remembered by turning "13" 90 degrees to its side (credit to Dr. Barone) and using the sideways "1" to remember polydactyly) and the sideways "3" to remember cleft lip.

PPx: N/A

MoD: Nondisjunction of chromosome 13

Dx: If quad screen positive, karyotype with amniocentesis

Tx/Mgmt: Surgery to correct cleft palate

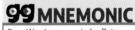

Medications During Pregnancy

A high-yield topic on the exam is how pregnant women should be counseled with respect to medication. These include the following recommendations:
- Diabetics should have good glycemic control and dietary counseling

- Women with hypothyroidism should have appropriate levothyroxine dosing
- Women receiving warfarin should switch to a different anticoagulant:
  - **Warfarin embryopathy:** facial abnormalities, optic atrophy, digital abnormalities, mental impairment, fetal bleeding → occurs if exposed early (6–12 weeks)
  - Later exposure to warfarin → central nervous system defects
  - High-risk situations (mechanical heart valve) still warrant warfarin use
  - **Low-molecular-weight heparins** are the most tolerated during pregnancy and most patients requiring anticoagulation should consider being switched to LMWH during the preconception period
- Women taking antiepileptics should approach their health care provider to consider switching/lowering dose:
  - Since NO antiepileptic drug has been proven to be safe, women should especially avoid **valproic acid,** which can cause neural tube defects and spina bifida
- Women taking isotretinoin for skin conditions should **not** get pregnant until 6 months after cessation:
  - Men and women must **register** for a national database known as iPLEDGE

GUNNER PRACTICE

1. A 6-month-old boy is brought into the doctor's office for examination. Although he is able to pull himself into a sitting position and can pass a toy back and forth between his hands, he appears to have trouble responding to who is talking to him and does not respond to his name. The patient feeds four or five times a day and passes greenish-brown stool. He has trouble sleeping and cries frequently. No complications were reported during pregnancy, although mom never made it to any of the prenatal visits. On exam, the patient is not anxious when the physician picks him up. He has a small head, wide-set eyes, and a smooth philtrum. What is the most likely diagnosis?
   A. Down syndrome
   B. Edward syndrome
   C. Patau syndrome
   D. Fetal alcohol syndrome (FAS)
   E. 22q11.2 deletion syndrome
2. A 33-year-old, gravida 3, para 3, woman gives birth to a newborn male at 39 weeks gestation. The mother had

been diagnosed with preeclampsia and gestational diabetes in previous pregnancies, but missed most of her
prenatal visits for this birth. She stated that she knew
what it took to deliver a healthy baby, and received much
of her advice from a private midwifery clinic. The exam
of the newborn finds a loud holosystolic murmur heard
at the left sternal border. His hands are balled into fists
with fingers overlapping. He is also found to have rocker
bottom feet. What screening test would have suggested
the newborn's diagnosis during the prenatal period?

A. Alpha fetal protein
B. Quad screen
C. beta-hCG and pregnancy-associated plasma
   protein A
D. First trimester ultrasound
E. Second trimester ultrasound

ANSWERS: What Would Gunner Jess/Jim Do?

1. WWGJD? A 6-month-old boy is brought into the doctor's office for examination. Although he is able to pull himself into a sitting position and can pass a toy back and forth between his hands, he appears to have trouble responding to who is talking to him and does not respond to his name. The patient feeds four or five times a day and passes greenish-brown stool. He has trouble sleeping and cries frequently. No complications were reported during pregnancy although mom never made it to any of the prenatal visits. On exam, the patient is not anxious when the physician picks him up. He has a small head, wide-set eyes, and a smooth philtrum. What is the most likely diagnosis?

Answer: D, Fetal alcohol syndrome

Explanation: The giveaway Buzz Word for fetal alcohol syndrome is a smooth philtrum. The chief complaint often is developmental delay, in which the patient is not meeting expected milestones. A 6-month-old infant, for instance, is expected to have stranger anxiety and be able to orient toward sound and name-calling. The patient in this question does neither, although he does meet the age-appropriate criteria for gross and fine motor movement (e.g., push to sit and transferring objects, respectively). Also, be wary of question stems in which the mother did not show up to prenatal visits. This means that risk factors, such as alcohol use, were likely not adequately communicated to mom. Patients with FAS will have mental retardation and ADHD-like symptoms as they progress through childhood.

A. Down syndrome → Incorrect. Patients with Down syndrome can have developmental delay but would have a simian crease in their palms as well as sandal-gapped toes. The characteristic facial feature is epicanthal folds and oblique palpebral fissures.

B. Edward syndrome → Incorrect. Patients with trisomy 18 have characteristic rocker bottom feet and overlapping fingers at birth and may have congenital heart defects at birth (e.g., VSD).

C. Patau syndrome → Incorrect. Patients with trisomy 13 have polydactyly and cleft lip.

E. 22q11.2 Deletion syndrome → Incorrect. Patients with 22q11.2 deletion syndrome have a constellation of symptoms and variable phenotypic presentation, but most typically on the shelf can appear to have micrognathia and low-set ears as well as conotruncal cardiac defects and an absent thymus (DiGeorge).

2. **WWGJD?** A 33-year-old, gravida 3, para 3, woman gives birth to a newborn male at 39 weeks gestation. The mother had been diagnosed with preeclampsia and gestational diabetes in previous pregnancies, but missed most of her prenatal visits for this birth. She stated that she knew what it took to deliver a healthy baby, and received much of her advice from a private midwifery clinic. The exam of the newborn finds a loud holosystolic murmur heard at the left sternal border. His hands are balled into fists with fingers overlapping. He is also found to have rocker bottom feet. What screening test would have suggested the newborn's diagnosis during the prenatal period?

Answer: B, Quad screen

Explanation: The newborn patient likely has a aneuploidy disorder called Edward syndrome as a result of three copies of chromosome 18. The chief screening test for trisomy 18 is a quad screen, which would show decreased AFP, hCG, estriol, and normal inhibin A. Quad screens are done at 15–20 weeks gestation and can help detect aneuploidy disorders that the baby may have.

A. AFP → Incorrect. Increased AFP suggests a neural tube defect while decreased AFP can be seen in Down, Edward, and Turner syndromes. It is part of the quad screen but cannot suggest trisomy 18 all on its own.

C. beta-hCG and pregnancy-associated plasma protein A → Incorrect. This is used to screen for Down syndrome in the first trimester, which is suggested by high beta-hCG and low PAPP-A levels.

D. First trimester ultrasound → Incorrect. The purpose of the first trimester ultrasound is for dating the fetus only (e.g., determining weeks of gestation). It cannot be used to screen for aneuploidy disorders.

E. Second trimester ultrasound → Incorrect. The purpose of the second trimester ultrasound is for dating the fetus. It cannot be used to screen for aneuploidy disorders.

Notes

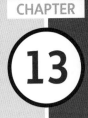
Disorders of the Skin and Subcutaneous Tissues

Angela Ester Ugorets, Jacob Charny, Hao-Hua Wu, Leo Wang, and Judy Chertok

Introduction

The Family Medicine shelf exam will often test your knowledge of dermatology with images, so it is important to know how to recognize and differentiate different skin diagnoses. To help you, we have included an image with each Dx below. Questions will focus on three skin cancers: melanoma, squamous cell carcinoma (SCC), and basal cell carcinoma (BCC). It is advantageous to know the Buzz Words and the risk factors, and be able to recognize these three on images. Benign skin conditions are also fair game, though less commonly tested, and again rely on your ability to recognize them in photographs and know their risk factors.

Benign Neoplasms, Cysts, and Other Skin Lesions

Actinic Keratosis (Also Called Solar Keratosis)

Buzz Words: scaly + sandpaper surface

Clinical Presentation: These are small, scaly, red lesions, considered pre-cancerous as they often lead to SCC if left untreated. They are common in fair-skinned individuals (light hair and eyes, those who are prone to sun burn, ex: northern European descent). They occur in sun-exposed areas: forehead (especially of balding men), face, neck, arms, back of hands, shoulders.

PPx: (1) Suncreen; (2) hat to cover scalp.

MoD: Cumulative damage from exposure to UV rays → mutations in keratinocytes → proliferation of abnormal keratinocytes

Dx: Physical exam with classic lesion findings

Tx/Mgmt:

1. Freeze with liquid nitrogen to prevent transformation into SCC
2. 5-flurouracil

Lipoma

Buzz Words: Fluctuant, smooth, doesn't go away

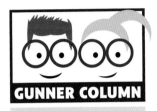

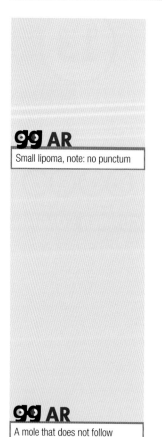

99 AR

Small lipoma, note: no punctum

99 AR

A mole that does not follow ABCDEs of Melanoma

Clinical Presentation: Lipoma is a benign overgrowth of fat cells (adipose) in a sac under the skin. They are easily confused with cysts. Like a cyst, a lipoma is also a fluctuant mass under the skin, but it stays the same size or grows slowly (doesn't come and go like a cyst), and it does not have a punctum. No redness, pain, or itching.

PPx: None

MoD: Unknown. May run in families

Dx: Physical exam

Tx/Mgmt:

1. Benign, no Tx/Mgmt necessary
2. Surgery

Pigmented Nevus (aka Melanocytic Nevus or Mole)

Buzz Words: Stable, symmetrical, unchanged, hair growing from them

Clinical Presentation: Pigmented nevus is a brown skin lesion that does not fit the ABCDEs of melanoma (explained under "Melanoma" section). If someone has many, they should all look the same on the same person. Some may be present at birth (congenital) but most are acquired. Congenital ones often have hair growing out of them, indicating that they are benign. They may change very gradually over the person's lifetime, such as becoming raised or fading. They do not change or grow rapidly.

PPx: None

MoD: Benign neoplasm formed mostly by melanocyte cells, which produce melanin and give moles their dark color.

Dx: Visualization under a dermatoscope

Tx/Mgmt: No Tx/Mgmt necessary, reassurance.

Seborrheic Keratosis

Buzz Words: Stuck on, pasted on, waxy, wart-like

Clinical Presentation: Seborrheic keratosis is the most common benign skin tumor. These are large, waxy, brown spots that appear on the body as a patient ages, and look as though they have been "stuck on" to the patient's skin. They can range in color from light brown to nearly black. They may look like a scab or something you could pick off, sometimes described as "wart-like" but are not true warts. They are sometimes itchy, but otherwise painless. Often there are many that appear on the back, chest, face.

PPx: None

MoD: Proliferation of keratinocytes (top layer of epidermis) that occurs in nearly everyone as they age. Mechanism not well understood.

Dx: Physical exam, can be confirmed with pathology report on biopsy.

Tx/Mgmt: Reassurance. These are benign.

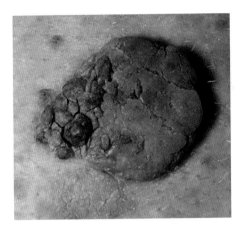

gg AR

Face

gg AR

Up close; appears "stuck on" skin

Malignant Neoplasms

Basal Cell Carcinoma (BCC)

Buzz Words: Pink, pearly, shiny, papule, telangectasias, rolled borders, upper lip

Clinical Presentation: BCC is the most common skin cancer; though it rarely metastasizes. Occurs in fair-skinned people, most often on sun exposed areas of head and neck: forehead, face, nose, *upper* lip, but can also occur on other sun-exposed areas like back of the hands, arms, shoulders, and back. Patient may complain of a changing lesion on face or neck that won't heal. It's often described as raised, pink, pearly, skin-colored papule with small telangectasias and rolled borders. It may ulcerate in the center and can be disfiguring. The patient is often someone who worked outdoors in the sun for many years (ex: farmer or soldier).

PPx: (1) Sunscreen (2) Wear a hat

MoD: Malignant overgrowth of basal cells, the deepest layer of cells of the epidermis, due to DNA damage from excessive exposure to UV light.

Dx: Biopsy with pathologic confirmation

Tx:

1. Electrodessication and Currettage ("EDC")
2. Surgical excision with 3-4mm margins
3. Mohs Micrographic Surgery (especially if large, on the face, or recurrent)

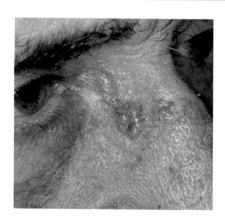

Note "pearly" lesion with telangectasias and rolled borders:

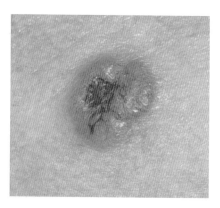

Squamous Cell Carcinoma (SCC)

Buzz Words: Ulcerating, non-healing, cigarette smoker, lower lip, sun exposure

Clinical Presentation: SCC is the second most common type of skin cancer. It's more likely to metastasize than BCC. Patients typically present with a new or growing lesion, may seem similar to a scab, that won't heal. It often bleeds intermittently and may itch. On exam, you will find an ulcerated sore that doesn't heal with a rough, scaly crust and/or borders. Risk factors include fair skin, sun exposure (ex: farmer, soldier), 3ʳᵈ degree burns, and cigarette smoking. Most likely to occur on sun exposed areas such as the face, especially ears, forehead, and *lower* lip (think of the cigarette resting on the lower lip creating an ulcer), arms, back of hands, shoulders, and back. Actinic Keratosis is a precancerous lesion that leads to SCC if not treated.

PPx: (1) sunscreen (2) Wear a hat

MoD: Malignant overgrowth of squamous cells, the layer of cells right above the basal cell (bottom) layer of the epidermis, due to DNA damage from excessive exposure to UV light.

Dx: Biopsy with pathologic confirmation

Tx:

1. Electrodessication and Currettage ("EDC")
2. Surgical excision with 4-6mm margins
3. Mohs Micrographic Surgery (especially if large, on the face, or recurrent)

SCC often arises on the lower lip, looks ulcerated:

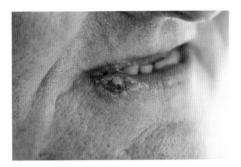

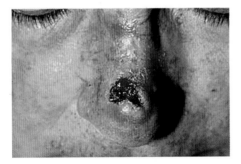

Melanoma

Buzz Words: Irregular, dark, rapidly growing, changing, asymmetric

Clinical Presentation:

The least common skin cancer, but the most deadly one. It tends to metastasize first to lymph nodes then to the brain, lungs, and bone (spine). It follows the ABCDE warning signs of melanoma:

A: Asymmetric

B: Borders—irregular, uneven

C: Color—has a variety of colors within one lesion, or unusual color (black, blue)

D: Diameter—over 6 mm (1/4 inch)

E: Evolving—patient may notice a rapid change in any of the ABCD

Melanomas may be itchy, crusty, or bleed. The depth of melanoma invasion is called Bresthlow thickness, and it determines the staging and prognosis. If melanoma is present on the palms of hands, soles feet, or under nail, it's called acral lentigenous melanoma. This form is more common in African-Americans.

PPx: (1) Incomplete recommendation from United States Preventative Services Task Force for screening. (2) Avoid excessive sun exposure.

MoD: Damage to melanocytes lead to out of control growth.

Dx: Biopsy with pathologic confirmation.

Tx/Mgmt: Wide excisional biopsy with 1 cm (or greater margins). Need pathologic confirmation of negative margins. Depending on the stage of the melanoma (0 through 4), may need sentinel lymph node biopsy, chemotherapy, immunotherapy, or radiation therapy.

gg AR

Irregular, asymmetric, growing, large, dark spot

Disorders of Sweat and Sebaceous Gland

Hidradenitis Suppurativa

Buzz Words: Draining tracts + armpits, groin, apocrine glands

Clinical Presentation: Hidradenitis suppurativa is characterized by clusters of clogged and draining cysts in bilateral armpits and/or in groin. They are very painful and often malodorous. After drainage, the cysts leave tracts to skin and create significant permanent scars and sometimes contractures. The disease most often occurs in young females. Patients are often embarrassed by these symptoms and this disease is often psychologically debilitating. Sometimes called "acne inversa."

PPx: None

MoD: Plugging of apocrine sweat glands for unknown reason.

Dx: Physical exam

Tx/Mgmt: No effective Tx/Mgmt known, however providers may (1) treat it like acne (e.g., topical clindamycin) or (2) perform incision and drainage ("I&D") on individual cysts that need to be drained for symptomatic relief

gg AR

Note scarring and sinus tracts

Acne Vulgaris

Buzz Words: Adolescent, facial eruption + whiteheads/blackheads comedones

Clinical Presentation: Acne vulgaris occurs when hair follicles become clogged with oil and dead skin cells, causing surrounding inflammation and redness. It can range from painless mild open comedones (called "blackheads"), moderate closed comedones (called "whiteheads"), or painful and disfiguring cystic lesions, which usually flare around the jawline and leave scars. They most often occur on the face, usually the forehead, on the nose, cheeks, chin, chest, back, and arms. While acne is medically benign, it can be psychologically disabling. It most commonly occurs during teenage years when androgen levels (testosterone) are high. Women's acne tends to flare during menstruation. Acne can also be a result of hyperandrogenism secondary to polycystic ovarian syndrome or Cushing's syndrome. Acne may run in families, and there is no proven connection between acne and diet or smoking.

PPx: Avoid touching or picking skin and overcleansing. Wear non-comedogenic make up.

MoD: Increased sebum production, proliferation of *Propionibacterium acnes* bacteria, plugging of hair follicles, and subsequent inflammation.

Dx:
1. Physical exam
2. Check testosterone level in women with acne, hirsutism, and irregular periods
3. Check morning cortisol level in suspected Cushing's syndrome or adrenal hyperplasia

Tx:
Varies based on extent and severity.
1. Topical regimen for mild acne includes benzoyl peroxide, retinoids, or clindamycin.
2. Systemic antibiotics, such as tetracycline, doxycycline, or minocycline are good for moderate acne in combination with topical Tx/Mgmt.
3. Isotretinoin ("Accutane") for severe and cystic acne:
   - Side effects of isotretinoin include elevated liver enzymes, depression, and teratogenicity (must make sure female patient is not pregnant).
   - Spironolactone is effective for women only.
   - Birth control may alleviate acne flares that correspond to a woman's menstrual cycle.

Open comedones (blackheads)

Pustules

Cystic acne, painful and disfiguring, leaves scars

Rosacea

Buzz Words: Red face + nasal hypertrophy + rhinophyma + flushing

Mild rosacea

Severe rosacea with pustules

Rhinophyma

Clinical Presentation: Rosacea is red flushing of the face, especially cheeks, nose, chin, and forehead, often triggered by temperature changes, sunlight, spicy or hot foods, alcohol, emotion, and stress. Rosacea occurs more often in middle age and post-menopausal Caucasian women, and is a lifelong condition once it starts. Some patients have pustules in addition to skin flushing. Severe rosacea can lead to a large, lobulated nose, called rhinophyma.

PPx: Avoid triggers, such as extreme changes in temperature (hot to cold or vice versa), direct sunlight (wear sunscreen or a hat), spicy or hot foods, and alcohol. However, avoiding triggers will not lead to remission.

MoD: Unknown; flushing may be related to dilated blood vessels under the skin surface.

Dx: Physical exam

Tx: Avoiding triggers. Topical metronidazole is the first-line for mild and moderate rosacea and an oral tetracycline antibiotic (e.g., doxycycline) is added for moderate to severe rosacea, which works by reducing inflammation. Some laser Tx/Mgmts may decrease capillaries.

Autoimmune and Allergic Skin Conditions

Psoriasis

Buzz Words: Silvery, scaly plaques + extensor surfaces + salmon-colored + itchy + pinpoint bleeding

Clinical Presentation: Psoriasis is an itchy, well-demarcated plaque with silver scale on top of an erythematous base, often described as "salmon-colored." These plaques generally occur on extensor surfaces like elbows and knees, and commonly on the scalp. In severe cases, it may cover the majority of the body. Lesions can also appear after an injury to the skin, known as "Koebner phenomenon." "Auspitz sign" refers to the pinpoint bleeding that occurs if the scale is picked off. Nail pitting is common. It can be associated with arthritis in up to 30% of patients. A more acute form known as guttate (drop-shaped) psoriasis can occur after upper respiratory or streptococcal infections. Psoriasis runs in families and is a lifelong condition.

PPx: N/A

MoD: Unknown, thought to be related to T-cell and keratinocyte dysfunction, causing rapid proliferation and maturation of keratinocytes.

Dx:
1. Physical exam
2. Pathologic confirmation from punch biopsy helpful if Dx is unclear
3. KOH preparation of scale can rule out fungal infection which may look similar

Tx/Mgmt:
1. Start with topical steroids, topical calcineurin inhibitors, or topical vitamin D for isolated lesions
2. Ultraviolet (UV) light for more widespread disease to induce and maintain remission
3. Systemic therapy consists of immunomodulation with methotrexate, mycophenolate mofetil, cyclosporine, tacrolimus, or injectable anti-tumor necrosis factor-alpha (TNFα) such as etanercept, infliximab, or adalimumab

99 AR

Psoriasis in scalp, note silver scale

99 AR

On extensor surfaces, classic location

99 AR

Psoriatic nail pitting (may only affect a few nails)

Atopic Dermatitis (aka Eczema)

Buzz Words: Pruritic + flexural surfaces + inside elbows, inside knee + "the itch that rashes"

Clinical Presentation: Chronic pruritic pink patches located in flexural areas, such as inside the knees and elbows, as well as on writs, hands and feet, the neck in older children and adults, or on the face (cheeks) of newborns and toddlers. The rash is poorly demarcated. Can become superinfected with herpes simplex virus (HSV), streptococci, or staphylococci as the barrier function of skin is compromised from repeated scratching. This scratching over time leads to patches of thickening and darkening of the skin, called lichen simplex chronicus. Associated with other atopic disorders, such as asthma, allergic rhinitis, and food allergies. Can be diffuse and severe, especially in children and young adults. The patient is likely to have dry skin throughout.

PPx: Frequent moisturization, sensitive skin care, avoiding triggers such as excessive or hot bathing and irritation.

MoD:
Unknown: some genetic component, hypothesized to be related to sterility of environment as a child—the more sterile the environment, the more likely to develop atopic dermatitis.

Dx:
1. Physical exam
2. Cultures for bacteria or viral polymerase chain reaction (PCR) helpful in diagnosing infection
3. Low threshold to test for allergies or asthma

Tx/Mgmt:
1. Topical corticosteroids intermittently during flares
2. Extensive disease may require systemic immunomodulation
3. Adjunctive antihistamines for pruritus
4. Antibiotic or antiviral therapy as needed for superinfection

Contact Dermatitis

Buzz Words: Exposures to nickel + dermatitis near belt buckle + Linear

Clinical Presentation: Erythematous, itchy eruption. Morphology can be vesicular, papular, plaque-like, or bullous. Occurs in the location of exposure, such as ear lobes for nickel allergy, lower abdomen for nickel belt buckle, or ankles for poison ivy contact. The eruptions are often linear from where the allergen swiped against the skin. A history of exposure to some irritant or chemical, such as latex, nickel, fragrances, or dyes is typical. The rash typically takes days or weeks to go away, as opposed to urticarial, which takes minutes to hours.

PPx: Determination and avoidance of the irritant or allergen

MoD: Type IV hypersensitivity reaction (cell-mediated)

Dx:
1. Clinical
2. Careful history and physical exam to determine irritant or allergen
3. Punch biopsy will show dermatitis, non-specific
4. Patch testing can elucidate allergen or irritant if trigger is unknown

Tx/Mgmt:
1. Avoidance of trigger
2. Topical corticosteroids
3. Adjunctive antihistamines for pruritus

GUNNER PRACTICE

1. A 60-year-old male comes to the doctor's office complaining of a "sunburn." He states that he was out in the sun gardening over the summer without putting on sunscreen or wearing a hat, and when he looks in the mirror, he sees some red marks on his forehead. For the past month, the red marks have not gone away. The patient is a construction worker who emigrated from Ireland 40 years ago. He takes hydrochlorothiazide for high blood pressure and metformin for diabetes. He smokes about a half a pack

of cigarettes per day. He has quit drinking ever since he was involved in an automobile accident with another drunk driver. At home, he lives with his wife. On exam, his forehead and the bridge of his nose have multiple scaly, erythematous lesions.

A. Seborrheic keratosis
B. Actinic keratosis
C. Melanoma
D. Herpes zoster
E. Contact dermatitis

ANSWERS: What Would Gunner Jess/Jim Do?

1. WWGJD? A 60-year-old male comes in to the doctor's office complaining of a "sunburn." He states that he was out in the sun gardening over the summer without putting on sunscreen or wearing a hat, and when he looks in the mirror, he sees some "red marks" on his forehead. For the past month, the "red marks" have not gone away. The patient is a construction worker who emigrated from Ireland 40 years ago. He takes hydrochlorothiazide for high blood pressure and metformin for diabetes. He smokes about a half a pack of cigarettes per day. He has quit drinking ever since he was involved in am automobile accident with another drunk driver. At home, he lives with his wife. On exam, his forehead and the bridge of his nose have multiple scaly, erythematous lesions. What is the most likely Dx?

Answer: B, Actinic keratosis

Explanation: The patient most likely has actinic keratosis due to his prolonged history of sun exposure as well as Buzz Words for these lesions (e.g., scaly erythematous lesions that appear at sun-exposed areas). His skin color (Caucasian from Ireland) and occupation (construction worker) have predisposed him the ill effects of chronic UV damage. Patients need to be treated with either liquid nitrogen freezing or 5-fluorouracil and monitored, as actinic keratosis can eventually lead to SCC.

A. Seborrheic keratosis → Incorrect. Seborrheic keratosis is also a proliferation of keratinocytes, but they present as dark brown in color and have a "stuck-on appearance" in the question stem.

C. Melanoma → Incorrect. Melanoma would typically appear as a black or brown macule that changes in size, shape, color, and depth over time.

D. Sunburn → Incorrect. Although it is tempting to choose this answer, a sunburn would not present as scaly erythematous lesions months after the initial insult (it most likely would have been healed).

E. Contact dermatitis → Incorrect. There was no mention of an object that made contact with the forehead and nose that would have led to contact dermatitis.

Diseases of the Musculoskeletal System and Connective Tissue

Hao-Hua Wu, Leo Wang, and Katherine Margo

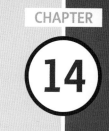

Introduction

Musculoskeletal disease can either encompass 5%–10% of the NBME Family Medicine shelf exam content or up to 15%–20% if the additional MSK module is added. As we suggested in the introduction, make sure you ask your clerkship director at the beginning of the rotation whether the MSK module will be included in the shelf, which is an additional 10 questions to the core 80-question exam. As is the case for other shelf exams, topics concerning pediatric orthopedics is very high yield for the Family Medicine shelf. This is because bones in the pediatric population heal more easily than adults, and unless there is damage to the physes, they can often get by with non-surgical treatment. Be sure to learn commonly tested disorders, such as nursemaid elbow and Osgood-Schlatter disease.

For the Family Medicine exam, you do NOT need to know the specifics of orthopedic procedures for the treatment of these diseases. Just know the general work-up and the Buzz Words for each disease.

This chapter is divided into (1) traumatic and mechanical disorders, (2) degenerative and metabolic disorders, (3) inflammatory disorders, (4) pediatric orthopedic disorders, and (5) Gunner practice.

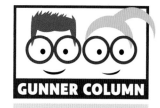

High-yield Pediatric Orthopedics video

Traumatic and Mechanical Disorders

Low Back Pain

Low back pain (LBP) is one of the most common complaints seen by a family medicine physician and, thus, a favorite topic of the shelf exam. In addition to learning about the differential for common causes of back pain, you may be asked about red flag symptoms as well as indications for ordering a lumbar X-ray.

According to the American Academy of Family Physicians, one should wait at least 6 weeks from the onset of back pain to get an X-ray. The only exception to that rule is if the following red flags are present:

1. Underlying medical illness with correlation to the spine (e.g., metastasis from cancer, spinal tuberculosis)
2. Bowel of bladder incontinence, saddle paresthesias, and other neurologic deficits that indicates direct damage to the spinal cord
3. Traumatic injury (e.g., falling out of a five-story window) or suspicion of fracture
4. Acute pain with point tenderness upon palpation of the spinous process, especially in the setting of a condition that predisposes to poor skeletal health (e.g., osteoporosis)
5. Fever or suspicion of infection

Lumbar Strain

Buzz Words: LBP immediately after physical activity + no history of LBP preceding + negative examination and work-up

Clinical Presentation: The shelf exam will most likely test you on the management of a lumbar strain. Remember that the recommendation is to resume normal activity (and not to rest) because data shows that the vast majority of LBP is self-limiting and could be made worse/stiff with immobility.

PPx:

(1) Avoid strenuous activity but do not advise complete immobility.

MoD: Mechanical stress (lifting something too heavy)

Dx:

1. No need to image unless there are red flags.
2. Rule out radiculopathy with straight leg raise.

Tx/Mgmt:

1. Nonsteroidal antiinflammatory drugs (NSAIDs).
2. Resume normal activity but no strenuous activity (resting without any activity does not improve LBP).

Spondylolysis

Buzz Words: LBP + exacerbated by activity (hyperextension) + Scotty dog sign

Clinical Presentation: Spondylolysis refers to phenomenon of fractures that appear in the interarticular portion of vertebral bone.

PPx:

(1) Avoid strenuous activity.

MoD: Repeated microtrauma, degenerative → fracture of pars interarticularis

Dx: X-ray to view pars intearticularis, oblique view to see the "Scotty dog sign," or a dog with a collar around neck

Tx/Mgmt: Conservative: NSAIDs, avoid physical activity.

Spondylolisthesis

Buzz Words: LBP + exacerbated by activity + vertebral body slipped forward on X-ray ± presence of spondylolysis

Clinical Presentation: Spondylolisthesis is the displacement of a vertebral body relative to the vertebral body beneath it.

PPx:

(1) Avoid strenuous activity.

MoD: Trauma, degenerative → slippage of superior vertebral body over inferior vertebral body

Dx: X-ray

Tx/Mgmt:

1. Conservative → NSAIDs, avoid physical activity
2. Cortisone
3. Spinal fusion

Spinal Stenosis

Buzz Words: LBP worse with activity + lower extremity pain + relieved by sitting and leaning forward (pushing a cart at the grocery store relieves back pain) + narrowing of canal on imaging + weakness/numbness of legs while walking → lumbar spinal stenosis

Neck pain/Upper back pain + radicular pain to arms + paresthesias/weakness of arm at compressed root → cervical spinal stenosis:

- May get UMN signs of lower extremity if cervical stenosis bad enough to cause myelopathy (spinal cord damage)

Weakness of upper extremity (LMN at level of cervical spine) + hyperreflexivity/Babinski sign of lower extremities (UMN signs below level of cervical spine → Advanced cervical spinal stenosis

Clinical Presentation: Spinal stenosis can be organized by region of spine. Cervical and lumbar regions are most common and is usually seen in the elderly.

PPx: None

MoD: Congenital; degenerative, osteophytes in the vertebral canal → narrowing of canal

- Osteophytes are bony spurs that form next to each other 2/2 chronic degeneration

Dx:

1. X-ray
2. MRI is most accurate

Tx/Mgmt:
1. Conservative → NSAIDs, avoid physical activity
2. Cortisone

Carpal Tunnel Syndrome

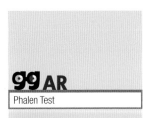

99 AR
Phalen Test

99 AR
Tinel Signs

99 AR
Carpal Tunnel Syndrome

Buzz Words: Pregnant + hyper/hypothyroid + repetitive hand work + pain in wrist/hand at night + numbness/tingling of fingers + positive Phalen or Tinel sign

Clinical Presentation: Because carpel tunnel syndrome is so easy to recognize, the shelf frequently likes to test on the **order of steps** for both diagnosis and treatment. Make sure you know each step well and in order.

PPx: Avoid repetitive wrist motion (e.g., extensive flexion and extension)

MoD: Compression of the median nerve secondary to swelling, often in the fibromuscular groove posterior to the medial epicondyle of the humerus:
- Can be secondary to diabetes, hypo/hyperthyroidism, acromegaly, pregnancy, dialysis-related amyloidosis

Dx:
1. Clinical
2. Wrist X-ray to rule out fractures/arthritis
3. **Nerve conduction studies** are the most likely to confirm the diagnosis (per NBME)
4. Electromyography ([EMG] if surgery is required)
5. Computed tomography/magnetic resonance imaging (MRI) only if EMG equivocal

Mgmt/Tx:
1. Rest and adjustment of aggravating activities
2. Splint
3. NSAIDs
4. Corticosteroid shots (effective in 80%–90% of patients but may return after months; should not be given >3 times a year)
5. Surgery (carpal tunnel release) as last resort (must have EMG beforehand)

Ankle Sprain

Sprain = injury to a ligament (e.g., ankle sprain means an injury to one of the ligaments of the ankle)

Strain = injury to a tendon

Buzz Words: Fall on a plantar flexed inverted foot + tenderness to the anterolateral ankle + can bear weight ≥4 steps + no medial malleolus tenderness + no lateral malleolus tenderness → likely ankle sprain with injury to the anterior talofibular ligament.

QUICK TIPS

Know the sequence of diagnostic and treatment steps! This is a common test question on the shelf (e.g., patient has already tried rest, splint, and NSAIDs. What is the next best treatment?).

QUICK TIPS

Difference between a sprain and a strain

Fall on a plantar flexed inverted foot + tenderness to the anterolateral ankle + unable to bear weight for four steps → indication for ankle X-ray based on Ottawa rules

Clinical Presentation: An ankle sprain is simply an injury to one of the many ligaments that stabilize the ankle. The ankle is the joint where the tibia and fibula meet with the talus. It is important to know the bones that articulate at the ankle joint because many of the ligaments are named after them!

The most commonly sprained ligament of the ankle, for instance, is the ATFL, which means it spans the talus and fibula on the anterolateral portion of the ankle (we know it is lateral because your fibula is always lateral to your tibia). Hopefully, now the first set of Buzz Words makes sense.

For the purposes of the shelf exam, it is very unlikely you will be asked to identify the specific ligament injured (although you could probably now identify the ATFL). Instead, you will likely be asked about the Ottawa ankle rules for referring a patient for an ankle X-ray, which states that an ankle X-ray series is required if there is pain in the malleolar zone AND one of these findings:

a. Inability to bear weight immediately after injury and in emergency department
b. Bony tenderness at posterior lateral malleolus
c. Bony tenderness at posterior medial malleolus

Remember, the medial malleolus is part of your tibia and the lateral malleolus is part of your fibula. The purpose of the Ottawa ankle rules is to cut down on unnecessary imaging.

PPx: (1) Ankle brace.

MoD: Variable but commonly application of a heavy force onto an inverted or everted foot

Dx:
1. Clinical (apply Ottawa ankle rules by palpating medial and lateral malleoli and asking patient to weight bear).
2. Ankle X-ray if and only if Ottawa criteria are met.

Tx/Mgmt:
1. Rest, ice compression and elevation (RICE)
2. NSAIDs
3. Ankle brace
4. Non-weight-bearing boot if high ankle sprain
5. Physical therapy (PT)
6. Operative management if refractory to conservative treatment

Ankle Anatomy

FOR THE WARDS

Two types of ankle sprains: high ankle sprain (injury to the syndesmosis, which is the ligament that connects the tibia and fibula) and low ankle sprain (injury to ligaments below the syndesmosis)

You may see different variations of the Ottawa ankle rule, including one that includes an age cutoff of 55 years of age. Those rules have since been updated from the original recommendation from 1992.

Rotator Cuff Tear

Buzz Words: Young athlete + pain with abduction and external rotation (throwing motion) + history of trauma or dislocation → likely rotator cuff tear

Older adult + pain with shoulder range of motion → likely rotator cuff tear

Supraspinatus → Abducts

Infraspinatus, Teres minor → Externally rotates

Subscapularis → Internally rotates

"Can remember the order because A-E-I are the first three vowels"

Clinical Presentation: Rotator cuff tears are commonly seen in athletes who play sports that involve throwing as well as patients >50 years old (secondary to degeneration over time). The purpose of the rotator cuff is to stabilize the shoulder and allow for several key movements, such as abduction, external rotation, and internal rotation.

Since rotator cuff injuries are straightforward to identify in a question stem, you will likely be asked where the lesion is (e.g., pain/weakness with abduction and empty-can test suggests supraspinatus tear) or what a physical exam finding means.

Commonly tested exam maneuvers are:

- Abduct arm to 90 degrees, angle forward 30 degrees, internally rotate thumb, and hold position (if painful when examiner exerts and downward force, then sign of supraspinatus tear: Jobe test or emptycan test)
- Flex shoulder to 90 degrees, flex elbow to 90 degrees, and forcibly internally rotate; if pain present, sign for impingement (Hawkins test)
- Raising hand between flexion and abduction all the way up while stabilizing ipsilateral scapula; if pain present, sign for impingement (Neer impingement test)

Of note, you do NOT need to memorize the eponyms. However, you do need to know what the exam maneuvers mean.

PPx: (1) Avoid repetitive motion of shoulder.

MoD: Traumatic or degenerative

Dx:

1. Clinical exam
2. X-ray
3. MRI

Tx/Mgmt:

1. Conservative: rest, PT, NSAIDs
2. Steroid injections
3. Surgery

Adhesive Capsulitis (aka Frozen Shoulder)

Buzz Words: Shoulder pain + stiffness + no other identifiable cause → adhesive capsulitis

Clinical Presentation: Adhesive capsulitis is pain or immobility of the shoulder due to **no identifiable cause.** This will most likely be one of the distractor answer choices on a question with a chief complaint of shoulder pain. It is associated with diabetes, thyroid disorders, and prolonged immobilization. Mostly self-limited but may require operative intervention if conservative measures fail.

PPx: (1) N/A

MoD: Idiopathic

Dx:

1. Physical exam (decreased range of motion and tenderness with motion)
2. Shoulder X-ray

Tx/Mgmt:

1. NSAIDs
2. PT
3. Steroid injection
4. Manipulation under anesthesia/surgery if conservative management fails

Anterior Dislocation of the Shoulder

Buzz Words: Athlete with severe pain + shoulder "popped" out of place + abduction and external rotation mechanism

Clinical Presentation: Severe pain, patients usually notice that the humeral head is out of place. Some athletes who are prone to this injury are gymnasts, football players, and wrestlers.

PPx: N/A

MoD: Forceful abduction, extension, and external rotation of the shoulder

Dx:

1. PE
2. X-ray
3. MRI:
   - Post reduction radiographs may show a posterior lateral humeral head impaction fracture (Hill-Sachs lesion). Sensation of the lateral deltoid region and the extensor surface of the proximal forearm should be verified, as they are altered with injury to the axillary nerve or the musculocutaneous nerve, respectively.

Tx/Mgmt: Immobilization after closed reduction:

- There is a high rate of recurrence, and rehabilitation focuses on strengthening the rotator cuff, deltoid, and pericapsular muscles.

Anterior shoulder dislocation video

Lateral Epicondylitis (Tennis Elbow)

Buzz Words: Tenderness in lateral elbow + plays tennis + pain with gripping activities + decreased grip strength

Clinical Presentation: Lateral epicondylitis is the inflammation of the extensor carpi radialis brevis (ECRB) at its origin. Occurs due to activities where there is repetitive pronation and supination while elbow is still in extension.

PPx: (1) Avoid tennis

MoD: Inflammation of the ECRB from repetitive overuse

Dx:

1. PE
2. X-ray to rule out fracture
3. MRI for definitive diagnosis

Tx/Mgmt:

1. RICE and physical therapy
2. NSAIDs
3. Surgery

Ligamentous Injuries to the Knee

Injuries to the knee are straightforward to understand if you know the anatomy and mechanism of injury. For instance, the four major ligaments that stabilize the knee are:

- Anterior cruciate ligament (ACL): resists anterior translation of tibia in relation to femur
- Posterior cruciate ligament (PCL): resists posterior translation of tibia in relation to femur
- Medial cruciate ligament (MCL): resists excessive valgus motion of the knee (valgus = force that moves distal end of extremity laterally; that is, the knee is in valgus if you hold the knee still with one hand and try to force the ankle to move laterally).

Thus, you should be able to identify the structure injured by the mechanism and exam presented in the question stem.

Unhappy triad: ACL tear, MCL tear and medial meniscal injury

Anterior Cruciate Ligament Tear

Buzz Words: Knee pain + popping sound heard + hemarthrosis + swelling + tibia translates anterior to femur (aka anterior laxity)

Clinical Presentation: ACL tears are a common sports injury seen particularly in athletes who do a lot of cutting/pivoting (e.g., female soccer players). You will likely only need to know the Buzz Words for the exam.

PPx: (1) Avoid cutting/pivoting motion.

MoD: Non-contact pivot injury

Dx:

1. PE (Lachman test, anterior drawer, pivot shift)
2. X-ray to rule out fracture
3. MRI for definitive diagnosis

Tx/Mgmt:
1. PT (does not automatically need surgery; can live functional life with just PT)
2. Surgery

Posterior Cruciate Ligament Tear

Buzz Words: Knee pain + tibia translating posterior to femur on exam + history of trauma to knee during flexion

Clinical Presentation: PCL tears are not as common as ACL tears, and will likely serve as a distractor answer choice for a chief complaint of knee pain.

PPx: (1) Avoid strenuous activity.

MoD: Traumatic force to proximal tibia with knee flexed

Dx:
1. PE (posterior drawer, neurovascular check, r/o dislocation)
2. X-ray to rule out fracture
3. MRI for definitive diagnosis

Tx/Mgmt:
1. PT (does not automatically need surgery; can live functional life with just PT)
2. Immobilization with brace
3. Surgery

Inflammatory Disorders

Septic Arthritis

Buzz Words: Acute onset of fever + exquisite joint tenderness with micromotion + swelling → septic arthritis

Clinical Presentation: Septic arthritis is the infection of a joint and requires emergent treatment. Classic presentation is a painful, swollen joint that exhibits pain even with slightest amount of motion (e.g., tenderness with micromotion). The hip is most commonly affected in younger children, whereas the knee is commonly affected in older children. Complications include avascular necrosis and cartilaginous damage.

PPx: An important risk factor of septic arthritis is gonorrhea, which can be seen in adolescents and adults who are at risk for sexually transmitted infections.

MoD: Hematogenous seeding of the synovial space. Less often, it can be the result of direct inoculation or extension from a contiguous focus. *Staphylococcus aureus* and *Streptococcus pyogenes* are the most common organisms. *Neisseria gonorrhoeae* may cause septic arthritis in adolescents.

Dx:
1. PE
2. Complete blood count (CBC)

3. ESR/CRP
4. Blood culture (positive in 30%–50% of cases)
5. Synovial fluid aspiration and culture (organisms and elevated WBC count)
6. Ultrasound may show fluid in joint

Tx/Mgmt:
1. Joint aspiration
2. Empiric IV antibiotics that cover Gram-positive organisms for 4–6 weeks

Gout

Buzz Words: Negatively birefringent crystals + recent large meal or alcohol consumption, swollen, red, and painful MTP joint of big toe (podagra) + tophus formation on external ear, olecranon bursa, or Achilles tendon → gout

Clinical Presentation: Gout, also known as monosodium urate crystal deposition disease, is caused by hyperuricemia, and is manifested by recurrent attacks of acute inflammatory arthritis, chronic arthropathy, accumulation of urate crystals, uric acid nephrolithiasis, most commonly in the MTP of the big toe. On the shelf, be able to distinguish this from other arthritides, as well as pseudogout. It is associated with underexcretion of uric acid (lead poisoning, alcoholism, excess red meat, seafood, beer, thiazides), overproduction of uric acid (Lesch-Nyhan syndrome, PRPP excess, increased cell turnover from leukemia or psoriasis treatment).

PPX: (1) Avoid excess red meats, seafood, alcohol, thiazides.

MoD: Prolonged hyperuricemia → tissue deposition of monosodium urate

Dx:
1. Uric acid levels (elevated)
2. CBC (absolute neutrophilic leukocytosis)
3. Must confirm with joint aspiration showing negatively birefringent MSU crystals

Tx/Mgmt:
1. Acute flare—NSAIDs (indomethacin, ibuprofen), glucocorticoids, colchicine
2. Chronic: xanthine oxidase inhibitors such as allopurinol, febuxostat

Pseudogout (Calcium Pyrophosphate Dihydrate Deposition Disease)

Buzz Words: Positively birefringent crystals + acute pain, redness, swelling, limited range of movement in joint + chondrocalcinosis → pseudogout

Clinical Presentation: In calcium pyrophosphate dihydrate deposition disease (CPPD), calcium pyrophosphate crystals deposit in joints, leading to inflammation. Deposition is common in elderly patients with degenerative joint disease, and increases with age and OA of the joints. In most cases, the cause of deposition is unknown, but joint trauma, hemochromatosis, hemosiderosis, hyperparathyroidism, and Bartter syndrome are risk factors. On the shelf, it is important to be able to distinguish the crystals of CPPD from gout.

PPx: Colchicine

MoD: Deposition of calcium pyrophosphate in tissues and cartilage (chondrocalcinosis)

Dx:
1. Chondrocalcinoisis on X-ray
2. Joint aspiration showing rhomboid crystals, weakly birefringent under polarized light

Tx/Mgmt:
1. NSAIDs, colchicine, glucocorticoids
2. Arthroscopic surgery

Degenerative and Metabolic Disorders

Patellofemoral Syndrome (Formerly Patellar Chondromalacia)

Buzz Words: Anterior knee pain + worse when descending stairs + patella in a lateral position

Clinical Presentation: Pain comes from contact of patella with the femur. Presents as knee pain that is difficult to localize, pain is often worse when climbing stairs, squatting, running, or sitting for prolonged periods. Physical examination may show the patella in a lateral position.

PPx: N/A

MoD: Joint malalignment and excessive use

Dx:
1. PE (medial patellar tenderness or pain with compression of the joint confirms the diagnosis in the absence of a significant effusion and other positive findings)
2. X-ray
3. MRI

Tx/Mgmt: Rest, stretching, and strengthening of the medial quadriceps

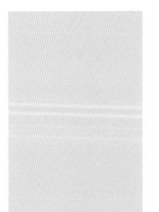

Intervertebral Disc Herniation

Buzz Words: Positive straight leg test + pain shooting down leg from back + paresthesias and weakness of lower extremity + unilateral → lumbar herniated disc

Positive Spurling test + pain shooting down arm + paresthesias and weakness of upper extremity + unilateral → cervical herniated disc

L3-L4 disc: weakness of knee extension, decreased patellar reflex

L4-L5 disc: weakness of dorsiflexion, difficulty in heel-walking

L5-S1 disc: weakness of plantarflexion, difficulty in toe-walking, decreased Achilles reflex

Disc Herniation: Cervical and Lumbar Radiculopathy

Disc	Root	Pain/Paresthesias	Sensory Loss	Motor Loss	Reflex Loss
C4-5	C5	Neck, shoulder upper arm	Shoulder	Deltoid, biceps, infraspinatus	Biceps
C5-6	C6	Neck, shoulder, lat. arm, radial forearm, thumb & index finger	Lat. arm, radial forewarm, thumb & index finger	Biceps, brachioradialis	Biceps, brachio-radialis, supinator
C6-7	C7	Neck, lat. arm, ring & index finger	Radial forearm, index & middle fingers	Triceps, extensor carpi ulnaris	Triceps, supinator
C7-T1	C8	Ulnar forearm and hand	Ulnar half of ring finger, little finger	Intrinsic hand muscles, wrist extensors, flexor dig profundus	Finger flexion
L3-4	L4	Anterior thigh, inner shin	Anteromedial thigh and shin, inner foot	Quadriceps	Patella
L4-5	L5	Lat. thigh and calf, dorsum of foot, great toe	Lat. calf and great toe	Extensor hallucis longus, floor dorsiflexion, inversion and eversion	None
L5-S1	S1	Back of thigh, lateral posterior claf, lat. foot	Posterolat. calf, lat. and sole of foot, smaller toes	Gastrocnemius, foot eversion	Achilles

Clinical Presentation: Due to desiccation of the annulus fibrosus, nucleus pulposus of intervertebral disc can herniate outward and compress the nerve of the superior vertebrae (e.g., intervertebral herniation of L4-5 will compress L4 root). Patients present with back pain and pain radiating into the legs (oftentimes the leg pain is worse than the back pain). Pain is often made worse by coughing, or sitting, and it may be relieved by standing up. Lumbar region is most commonly affected. Patient may lean toward unaffected side to relieve pressure on the spinal cord.

PPx: N/A

MoD: Tear in the annulus fibrosus, which allows protrusion of the nucleus pulposus. Unlike adults, in children it is mostly caused by repetitive activity, and rarely by trauma.

Dx:
1. PE
2. X-ray
3. MRI:
   - Radiographs show loss of lumbar lordosis due to muscle spasm, sometimes a mild lumbar scoliosis, as well as loss of intervertebral disc height
   - MRI is the best study to establish diagnosis

Tx/Mgmt:
1. Rest and PT
2. NSAIDs
3. Steroid injections
4. Surgery

Osteoarthritis

Buzz Words: Joint crepitus with motion + pain worse with motion + joint stiffness after inactivity + osteophyte enlargement of DIP joints (Heberden nodes), PIP joints (Bouchard nodes) + joint space narrowing on radiographs → OA

Clinical Presentation: Osteoarthritis is the most common chronic degenerative condition of the joints and occurs due to non-inflammatory breakdown of articular cartilage. This results in pain, stiffness, and loss of joint mobility, most commonly in hip, knee, back, PIP, and DIP. The pain is worse with use of the joint and improves with rest. Radiographic features include joint space narrowing, subchondral sclerosis, osteophyte formation, and subchondral cysts.

PPx: Maintain healthy weight, engage in physical activity

MoD: Non-inflammatory progressive articular cartilage degeneration at weight-bearing joints: femoral head, knee, cervical and lumbar vertebrae

Dx:
1. PE
2. X-ray

Tx/Mgmt:
1. Heat, decreased weight bearing, PT
2. Use of a cane and brace
3. Analgesics (NSAIDs)
4. Steroid injection, versus viscosupplementation versus surgery (arthroplasty aka joint replacement)

Avascular Necrosis of Femoral Head

Buzz Words: Corticosteroids + excessive alcohol intake + recent total hip replacement + crescent sign (subchondral radiolucency)

Clinical Presentation: Avascular necrosis is due to death of bone tissue due to a lack of blood supply, resulting in arthritis. On the shelf, remember the risk factors for avascular necrosis and be able to identify its appearance on radiograph.

PPx: N/A

MoD: Compromise of bone vasculature 2/2 multiple predisposing etiologies

Dx:
1. Clinical (H&P)
2. MRI for early detection due to high sensitivity
3. Anterior-posterior and frog-leg lateral films showing mild density changes, or pathognomonic crescent sign (subchondral radiolucency) in later phases

Tx/Mgmt:
1. Supportive (non-operatively)
2. Surgery—core decompression
3. If refractory, then total hip replacement

Osteopenia/Osteoporosis

Buzz Words: Elderly lady + hip fractures

Clinical Presentation: Osteopenia and osteoporosis are diseases that fall on a spectrum of decreased bone mineral density, where osteopenia can sometimes be considered to be a precursor to osteoporosis. To be diagnosed with osteopenia, the bone mineral density T-score falls between −1.0 and −2.5, while to be diagnosed with osteoporosis, the bone mineral density T-score is < −2.5. Osteopenia is a sign of normal aging, in contrast to osteoporosis, which is present in pathologic aging.

It is important to also realize that osteoporosis in question stems may refer to secondary osteoporosis, caused by excess steroids, Cushing syndrome, hyperthyroidism, long-term heparin, hypogonadism, or vitamin D deficiency.

PPx: (1) Screen in women ≥65 years old or in younger women whose fracture risk is equal to that of a 65-year-old woman; USPSTF have no recommendations for screening in men. (2) Calcium, vitamin D, weight-bearing exercise, smoking cessation.

MoD: Rate of bone resorption exceeds rate of bone formation after peak bone mass is attained. Associated with low estrogen (menopause), calcium/vitamin D deficiency, decreased physical bone mass, hypogonadism, hyperthyroidism, smoking, alcohol abuse, corticosteroids, prolonged heparin use, Cushing syndrome

Dx:

1. DEXA scan:

Osteopenia: DEXA bone mineral density T-score between −1.0 and −2.5

Osteoporosis: DEXA bone mineral density T-score < −2.5

Tx/Mgmt:

1. Non-pharmacologic—adequate calorie, calcium, and vitamin D, weight-bearing exercise, smoking cessation, reduce EtOH intake
2. For established osteoporosis or high-risk osteopenia, bisphosphonates
3. PTH therapy for 24 months

Dupuytren Contracture

Buzz Words: Painless stiffness of fingers + nodules on palmar fascia + contractures (baseline flexion at MCP or PIP joint) + palpable cord running longitudinally in subcutaneous tissue which puckers the skin and limits extension

Clinical Presentation: Dupuytren contracture is a contracture of the proliferated longitudinal bands of the palmar aponeurosis lying between the skin and flexor tendons in the distal palm and fingers, most commonly in the ring and small fingers. It begins as a nodule and progresses to fibrous bands, with contracture of the fingers. Associated with diabetes, cigarettes, alcohol use, repetitive hand use, familial history of contracture.

PPX: N/A

MoD: Slowly progressive fibroblastic proliferation and disorderly collagen deposition with fascial thickening

Dx: Clinical

Tx/Mgmt:
1. Glove with padding, or modifying tools with cushions
2. Glucocorticoid injection (triamcinolone acetonide and lidocaine)
3. Collagenase injection
4. Surgery (fasciotomy)

Pediatric Orthopedic Disorders
Legg-Calvé-Perthes Disease

Buzz Words: 4- to 10-year-old boy + insidious hip/knee pain with painful limp → Perthes disease

Clinical Presentation: Legg-Calvé-Perthes disease is idiopathic avascular necrosis of the proximal femoral epiphysis and affects children from 4 to 10 years of age. It can begin as painless but will progress to a mildly painful limp, usually related to activity. Decreased internal rotation and abduction of the hip. Pain may be referred to the knee or the groin. Has been found to be associated with attention deficit hyperactivity disorder and delayed bone age. High yield for the Pediatrics shelf.

PPx: N/A

MoD: Temporary interruption of blood flow to the femoral epiphysis, causing avascular necrosis. Etiology is unknown.

Dx:
1. PE
2. X-ray: AP and frogleg lateral views
3. Bone scan
4. MRI with contrast
5. Arthrogram:
   - Affected femoral head appears small, shows sclerotic bone and widened joint space. Presence of a crescentic subchondral fracture in the femoral head is termed the "crescent sign."

Tx/Mgmt:
1. Non-weight bearing
2. PT
3. NSAIDs
4. Surgery:
   - Principle of treatment is to contain the femoral head within the acetabulum, which prevents deformation of the femoral head.

Developmental Dysplasia of the Hip

Buzz Words: Joint laxity/clicking + breech delivery + positive Barlow and Ortolani maneuvers

gg AR
Developmental Dysplasia of the Hip video

Clinical Presentation: Asymptomatic in infants, careful examination will reveal hip dislocation using Ortolani and Barlow maneuvers. In infants older than 3 months of age, the dislocation can become relatively fixed, and the Galeazzi test should be used. Increased risk in the newborn with breech presentation, positive family history, females, and first-born children.

PPx: The typical physical examination of the newborn includes the use of Ortolani and Barlow maneuvers, this is because an earlier detection of this condition leads to a better clinical outcome.

MoD: Abnormality in stability or shape of the femoral head and acetabulum

Dx:

1. Physical examination demonstrating hip instability, asymmetry, or limited abduction
2. Imaging may be helpful to confirm the diagnosis, ultrasound is used for infants younger than 6 months of age because the hip and pelvis are not yet ossified at that age
3. AP radiographs may be used in infants older than 6 months of age

Tx/Mgmt:

1. Pavlik harness is recommended for infants younger than 6 months
2. While reduction under anesthesia is usually necessary, the diagnosis is not made until after 6 months of age
3. Monitoring with regular hip radiographs until the child is skeletally mature is necessary

Osgood-Schlatter Disease

Buzz Words: 12-year-old boy + basketball player + **pain over the tibial tuberosity**

Clinical Presentation: Osgood-Schlatter disease is inflammation of the patellar tendon at the insertion of the tibial tubercle (e.g., apophysitis). Patient presents with swelling of the tibial tuberosity with pain and tenderness over the tibial tubercle that is exacerbated with activity and relieved with rest. Most common in 10- to 15-year-old boys who participate in sports involving repetitive jumping. Usually asymmetric, but can be bilateral.

PPx: N/A

MoD: (1) Overuse of the extensor mechanism of the patella, causing traction apophysitis at the insertion of the patellar tendon to the proximal tibia.

Dx: Clinical; imaging not necessary unless the patient has unusual complaints

Tx/Mgmt:
1. Activity modification, rest, ice after exercise
2. A protective pad can be used over the tibial tubercle to protect from direct trauma
3. Severe cases, immobilization of the joint may be necessary

Slipped Capital Femoral Epiphysis

Buzz Words: Overweight 12 year old + dull pain in the hip that worsens with physical activity

Clinical Presentation: Non-radiating, dull, aching pain in the hip, groin, thigh, or knee that causes an altered gait. Internal rotation, flexion, and abduction are usually decreased in the affected hip. Pain is usually increased with physical activity. Risk factors include obesity, hypothyroidism, hypopituitarism, and renal osteodystrophy. Very high yield for the Pediatrics shelf.

PPx: N/A

MoD: Likely a combination of mechanical and endocrine factors.

Dx:
1. PE
2. AP and frog-leg lateral radiographs reveal posterior displacement of the femoral epiphysis. Earliest changes include widening and irregularity of the physis, with thinning of the proximal epiphysis

Tx/Mgmt: The goal is to prevent further progression of the slip and to stabilize the physis. This is done by pinning the epiphysis with a single, large screw. Osteonecrosis and chondrolysis are the two most serious complications.

Scoliosis

Buzz Words: Asymmetry of the shoulders or iliac crests + bump in the back while bending down

Clinical Presentation: Scoliosis presents as asymmetry of shoulder height, scapular position, and iliac crests. Adam's forward bending test is performed by having the child bend forward from the waist, while the examiner looks for a lower back prominence representing posterior displacement of the spine. Scoliosis is typically painless, and the presence of pain may indicate an underlying disorder that should be investigated.

PPx: Scoliosis screening of questionable benefit

MoD: Most cases are idiopathic; however, it can be caused by leg-length discrepancy, neuromuscular disorders, vertebral anomalies, connective tissue disorders, or genetic syndromes.

Dx:
1. PE
2. X-ray: PA and lateral radiographs of the spine are used to calculate the Cobb angle, which measures the angle between the superior and inferior vertebrae tilted into the curve

Tx/Mgmt:
1. No treatment for mild disease
2. Exercise
3. Bracing
4. Surgery

Subluxation of the Radial Head (Nursemaid Elbow)

Buzz Words: Child <6 year old + arm pulled by caretaker + pain with flexed elbow

Clinical Presentation: Pain and persistence of elbow flexion even though the patient's hand function is normal. Usually presents after a strong, pulling force is exerted on the arm in patients younger than 6 years of age. Extremely high yield for the Family Medicine shelf.

PPx: N/A

MoD: Sudden, strong, upward pulling of the arm causing rapid extension of the elbow. This causes a dislocation of the annular ligament into the joint and between the radial head and the humerus.

Dx: H&P:
- Radiographs are usually normal because the subluxation is usually inadvertently reduced by the technician while positioning the arm for imaging.

Tx/Mgmt: **Rotation of the forearm into supination while pressuring the radial head.** A successful reduction can usually be felt as a click, after which the child recovers movement of the joint and the pain is relieved.

GUNNER PRACTICE

1. A 12-year-old boy is brought into the clinic by his mother due to right knee pain. The patient states that the pain is worse after basketball practice and that the pain started 2 weeks ago. His mother states that he had symptoms of a cold a week before that. Physical examination reveals pain and tenderness in the tibial tubercle. What is the next step in the management of this patient?
    A. Obtain a plain radiograph of the right knee to visualize lateralization of the patella
    B. Immobilization of the right knee using a cast

C. Activity modification, ice after exercise, and NSAIDs

D. Surgical intervention

2. A 2-year-old female presents with irritability and limping on the right leg that started a day ago. The patient's temperature is 38.7°C(101.6°F), her heart rate is of 90 beats per minute, and her respiratory rate is 26 breaths per minute. Lab results show a white blood cell (WBC) count of 20,000/mm^3 and an elevated ESR. Physical examination reveals pain with movement of the right hip, which the patient maintains flexed, abducted, and externally rotated. Which of the following is a major complication if the condition is not treated on time?

A. Avascular necrosis of the joint

B. Slipped capital femoral epiphysis

C. Involvement of other joints

D. Dislocation of the hip

3. A newborn female with breech presentation was delivered by a 25-year-old primigravida via Cesarean section and is being examined by a pediatrician. The mother told the pediatrician that she did not have access to regular prenatal care. During the physical examination, the pediatrician notices a palpable clunk when pressure in the posterior direction is applied to the flexed and abducted hip, this is followed by another palpable clunk with hip abduction. The rest of the physical examination is normal. Which of the following is the best course of action for this patient?

A. Immobilization of the hip using a cast

B. Radiograph of the hip joint

C. Surgical intervention

D. Repeat physical examination in 2 weeks

Notes

ANSWERS: What Would Gunner Jess/Jim Do?

1. WWGJD? A 12-year-old boy is brought into clinic by his mother due to right knee pain. The patient states that the pain is worse after basketball practice and that the pain started 2 weeks ago. His mother states that he had symptoms of a cold a week before that (distractor). Physical examination reveals pain and tenderness in the tibial tubercle. What is the next step in the management of this patient?

Correct answer: C, Activity modification, ice after exercise, and NSAIDs

> Explanation: This patient has a classic clinical presentation of Osgood-Schlatter disease, which is caused by repetitive stress of the insertion of the patellar tendon in the tibial tubercle. This disease presents with pain and tenderness in the tibial tubercle, in patients between 10 and 15 years of age, which is worse with exercise. Activity modification, ice after exercise, and NSAIDs are enough to manage this condition, although it may take between 12 and 18 months to completely resolve.

> A. Obtain a plain radiograph of the right knee to visualize lateralization of the patella → Incorrect. The diagnosis of Osgood-Schlatter disease is clinical, and plain radiographs may reveal irregularities of the tubercle ossification center. Lateralization of the patella may be visualized in patello-femoral syndrome.

> B. Immobilization of the right knee using a cast → Incorrect. Activity modification is usually sufficient and immobilization of the knee is reserved for severe cases.

> C. Surgical intervention → Incorrect. Surgical intervention is not necessary to treat Osgood-Schlatter disease.

2. WWGJD? A 2-year-old female presents with irritability and limping on the right leg that started a day ago. The patient's temperature is 38.7°C(101.6°F), her heart rate is 90 beats per minute, and her respiratory rate is of 26 breaths per minute. Lab results show a WBC count of 20,000/mm³ and an elevated ESR. Physical examination reveals pain with movement of the right hip, which the patient maintains flexed, abducted, and externally rotated. Which of the following is a major complication if the condition is not treated on time?

Correct answer: A, Avascular necrosis of the joint

> Explanation: This patient presents with a fever, hip pain with limited range of motion, elevated WBC count,

and elevated ESR—all of which are classically present in a young child with septic arthritis. One of the classic complications of untreated septic arthritis is avascular necrosis of the head of the femur and destruction of the hip joint.

B. Slipped capital femoral epiphysis → Incorrect. This condition classically presents in overweight toddlers or adolescents. The elevated ESR and WBC count would not be present.

C. Involvement of other joints → Incorrect. This is not a classic complication of septic arthritis.

D. Dislocation of the hip → Incorrect. This is not a classic complication of septic arthritis.

3. WWGJD? A newborn female with breech presentation was delivered by a 25-year-old primigravida via cesarean section and is being examined by a pediatrician. The mother told the pediatrician that she did not have access to regular prenatal care. During the physical examination, the pediatrician notices a **palpable clunk when pressure in the posterior direction is applied to the flexed and abducted hip, this is followed by another palpable clunk with hip abduction. The rest of the physical examination is normal. Which of the following is the best course of action for this patient?**

Answer: D, Repeat physical examination in 2 weeks

Explanation: The maneuvers described in the physical examination are the Ortolani and Barlow maneuver, which are useful to detect developmental dysplasia of the hip. This condition is more common in first-born females. Screening with these maneuvers is recommended on all newborns, since an early diagnosis can reduce the risk of necessary surgical intervention. In most cases, the hip stabilizes within the first 2 weeks of life without the need for surgical intervention. Persistence of hip instability beyond that point warrants referral to an orthopedic surgeon.

A. Immobilization of the hip using a cast. → Incorrect. Children younger than 6 months who require treatment are immobilized using a Pavlik harness; this keeps the hip abducted and flexed and is the best initial treatment.

B. Radiograph of the joint → Incorrect. Imaging may be useful in the diagnosis of developmental dysplasia of the hip; however, in patients younger than 6 months, ultrasound is preferred.

C. Surgical intervention → Incorrect. Surgical reduction of the hip is not the preferred treatment in patients younger than 6 months of age.

Endocrine and Metabolic Disorders

Chevonne Parris-Skeete, Leo Wang, Hao-Hua Wu, and Katherine Margo

15

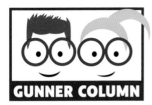

GUNNER COLUMN

Introduction

Endocrine and metabolic diseases encompass a vast array of conditions that affect the body's ability to maintain homeostasis. Although many of these conditions are seen frequently in practice, these questions only make up about 5%–10% of the Family Medicine shelf exam. As such, pay heavy attention only to the high-yield topics in this section. The most important disease in this chapter is **diabetes**.

Diabetes and Other Disorders of the Endocrine Pancreas

Type I Diabetes

Buzz Words:

Polyuria/polydipsia/nocturia + fatigue/weight loss

Clinical Presentation:

More common form of childhood diabetes. These patients present with typical findings like polyuria and polydipsia, sometimes with enuresis. Remember that these patients can be treated with insulin.

PPx:

N/A

MoD:

Autoimmune, lymphocytic destruction of pancreatic islet cells leads to deficient production in insulin. Can be overcome by supplementing insulin.

Dx:

1. Fasting glucose >126 g/dL
2. Blood sugar—random blood sugar >200 g/dL with symptoms
3. HbA1c > 6.5%

Tx/Mgmt:

1. Insulin:
   a. Every 3 months, check HbA1c (goal <7%).
   b. Every year, check urinalysis for microalbuminuria (if positive, start on angiotensin-converting enzyme [ACE] inhibitor or angiotensin receptor blockers [ARBs]), serum blood urea nitrogen (BUN), and creatinine (monitor for diabetic nephropathy), eye

screening with ophthalmologist (monitor for diabetic retinopathy), and cholesterol levels (if low-density lipoprotein [LDL] >100, start a statin).
c. Every visit, check blood glucose, blood pressure (if >130/80, start ACE inhibitor or ARB), feet (for ulcers).

Type II Diabetes

Buzz Words:
hyperglycemia + polyuria + polydipsia + polyphagia + nocturia

Clinical Presentation:
Unlike type I, type II diabetes is characterized predominately by insulin resistance. Diabetes is the leading cause of chronic kidney disease (CKD), non-traumatic lower limb amputations, and new cases of blindness among adults in the USA. The leading cause of death among diabetics is coronary artery disease.

Patients will often complain of frequent urination, plus excessive thirst and hunger (polyuria, polydipsia, polyphagia).

PPx:
(1) The United States Preventative Services Task Force recommends screening for abnormal blood glucose in patients 40–70 years old who are also overweight/obese. Screening occurs every 3 years with normal blood glucose level. (2) Weight control and exercise for prevention.

MoD:
Inadequate insulin secretion for serum glucose levels and insulin resistance in target tissues—particularly adipose tissue and skeletal muscle

Dx:
Abnormal results usually require a confirmatory test, unless the patient also presents with the Buzz Word symptoms:
a. Fasting [glucose] (mg/dL) ≥126
b. Oral glucose tolerance testing 2-hour [glucose] (mg/dL) ≥200
c. HbA1c (%) ≥6.5

Tx/Mgmt:
Patient education is very important, in addition to the following:
a. Diet and lifestyle modification
b. Metformin (contraindicated in CKD)
c. Sulfonylureas (can cause severe hypoglycemia)
d. Thiazolidinediones (cardiotoxic)
e. Incretin-based (weight loss)

QUICK TIPS
Many patients will have a transient decrease in insulin requirements after they first take it due to recovering function for the first 2 years of treatment; this is known as a honeymoon period.

QUICK TIPS
Somogyi phenomenon is when patients have hyperglycemia in the morning due to too much insulin taken before bed. Too much insulin at night → hypoglycemia → compensatory mechanisms → hyperglycemia in morning. LOWER insulin in these patients before bed.

99 AR
Diabetes Pathophysiology

QUICK TIPS
Treatment goal HbA1c ≤ 7%

QUICK TIPS
Metformin is the gold standard for initial pharmacologic therapy.

QUICK TIPS
Metformin is the only antidiabetic therapy shown to decrease cardiovascular risk and all-cause mortality.

f. Insulin (typically used after the failure of oral or other non-insulin therapies)

According to AAFP, Type II diabetes targets should be re-assessed every 3 months. Additional therapies are warranted if initial metformin treatment is not adequate.

Thyroid and Parathyroid Disorders

Hyperthyroidism

Graves Disease

Buzz Words:

heat intolerance + weight loss + palpitations + tremors + ophthalmopathy + pretibial myxedema + diffusely enlarged thyroid gland

Clinical Presentation:

Graves is the most common cause of hyperthyroidism. Patients may complain of heat intolerance, weight loss, palpitations, tremors, diarrhea, anxiousness, and oligomenorrhea.

PPx:

N/A

MoD:

Production of thyroid-stimulating immunoglobulins that bind to and activate the thyroid stimulating hormone (TSH) receptor, facilitating thyroid hormone secretion and gland growth

Dx:

1. Low TSH, high T4 and T3
2. Diffusely enlarged thyroid gland on uptake scan

Tx/Mgmt:

1. β-blockers
2. Propylthiouracil (PTU; used during first trimester in pregnant women)
3. Methimazole (MTZ; teratogenic—for pregnant women, used only in the second and third trimesters)
4. Radioactive iodine ablation (can cause postablative hypothyroidism)

Hypothyroidism

Autoimmune Thyroiditis (Hashimoto Thyroiditis)

Buzz Words:

Cold intolerance + fatigue + weight gain despite poor appetite + constipation + dry skin + menorrhagia + myalgias + lymphocytes + inflammation + autoantibodies

Clinical Presentation:

Autoimmune thyroiditis is the most common cause of primary hypothyroidism in developed countries; iodine deficiency is the primary cause in developing countries

PPx:

N/A

MoD:

Lymphocytic infiltration and inflammatory destruction
result in fibrosis and impaired gland function.

Dx:

1. Complete blood count (CBC)/basic metabolic panel
2. Elevated TSH, low T4 and T3

Tx/Mgmt:

Hormone replacement with levothyroxine

Hyperparathyroidism

Buzz Words:

Bone pain + renal stones + gastrointestinal (GI) disturbances
+ central nervous system (CNS) changes + weakness

Clinical Presentation:

Patients with hyperparathyroidism present with bone pain,
constipation, nausea, depression, lethargy, seizures,
weakness, and fatigue (signs/symptoms of hypercalcemia). Can be associated with MEN 1.

PPx:

N/A

MoD:

Elevated parathyroid hormone (PTH) secretion, resulting
in increased ionized serum calcium:
1. Primary: autonomous overproduction of PTH,
usually the result of an adenoma or hyperplasia of
parathyroid tissue
2. Secondary: compensatory hypersecretion of PTH in
response to hypocalcemia
3. Tertiary: persistent hypersecretion of PTH even after
the cause of the prolonged hypocalcemia is corrected

Dx:

Elevated PTH

Tx/Mgmt:

Parathyroidectomy

Adrenal Disorders

Hypercortisolism (Cushing Syndrome)

Buzz Words:

Hypertension + weight gain + truncal obesity + moon facies
+ buffalo hump + hyperglycemia + easy bruising + striae +
osteoporosis + mental disturbances + recurrent infections

Clinical Presentation:

Patient's with Cushing syndrome complain of decreased
libido, weight gain, menstrual changes, hirsutism,
weakness.

QUICK TIPS

Myxedema coma is severe hypothyroidism characterized by hypo-
thermia, bradycardia, hypotension,
AMS, and multisystem organ
failure → medical emergency

MNEMONIC

—painful bones, renal stones,
abdominal groans, psychic moans

QUICK TIPS

Parathyroid adenoma is the
most common cause of primary
hyperparathyroidism.

QUICK TIPS

Secondary hyperparathyroidism
is most commonly due to chronic
renal failure.

QUICK TIPS

Most are diagnosed incidentally
because serum calcium levels are
assessed on routine blood tests.

QUICK TIPS

Most common cause of hypercor-
tisolism is exogenous steroids.

PPx:
N/A
MoD:
(1) ACTH-dependent: elevated levels of glucocorticoids due to increased ACTH secretion (2) ACTH-independent: elevated levels of glucocorticoids in the absence of ACTH secretion

Dx:
24-hour urine free-cortisol level (increased); loss of normal diurnal patter of cortisol secretion:
    a. ACTH-dependent: elevated cortisol, elevated ACTH
    b. ACTH-independent: elevated cortisol, low ACTH

Tx/Mgmt:
1. Resection
2. Radiation therapy

Primary Chronic Adrenocortical Insufficiency (Addison Disease)

Buzz Words:
hyperpigmentation of the skin + weakness + GI complaints + hypotension

Clinical Presentation:
Presents as progressive weakness, easy fatigability, and darkening of the skin. Can be seen in people with other autoimmune conditions, such as type I diabetes mellitus.

PPx:
N/A
MoD:
Progressive destruction of the adrenal cortex, resulting in decreased levels of cortisol and aldosterone

Dx:
High ACTH, low cortisol, low aldosterone:
    a. ACTH stimulation test: cortisol levels will not rise following intravenous ACTH

Tx/Mgmt:
Hormone replacement

Pheochromocytoma

Buzz Words:
Paroxysmal hypertension + tremor + headache + palpitation

Clinical Presentation:
Presents as intermittent headaches, palpitations, tremor, and GI complaints. Can be associated with MEN 2, von Hippel-Lindau syndrome, and neurofibromatosis 1.

PPx:
N/A

MoD:

Neoplasm, which synthesizes and releases
   catecholamines

Dx:

1. Increased fractionated metanephrines in a 24-hour
   urine collection
2. Confirmatory computed tomography or magnetic resonance imaging for localization

Tx/Mgmt:

Adrenergic blockers followed by surgical resection

GUNNER PRACTICE

1. A 45-year-old man comes in for a routine health exam. He
   was last seen 3 years ago, when he was diagnosed with
   hyperlipidemia. He was placed on atorvastatin, but admits
   to not being compliant with his cholesterol medication. He
   notes increased urinary frequency, most notably at night.
   He denies changes in his vision or chest pain. However,
   he has recently noticed his feet have been "feeling funny."
   The patient is a truck driver and mainly eats on the road.
   On physical exam, his blood pressure is 132/84, respiration is 16, pulse is 95, and temperature is 98.7 °F. Body
   mass index is 32. Distal pulses are intact. A monofilament
   test showed decreased sensation in his right toes. What is
   the most likely cause of this patient's complaints?
   A. Urinary incontinence
   B. Diabetes mellitus
   C. Peripheral vascular disease
   D. Psychogenic polydipsia
2. A 38-year-old administrative assistant comes into the
   office with a complaint of increasing anxiety. She states
   she was recently promoted to administrative assistant
   in a law firm and, as a result, has taken on much more
   responsibility. At times she feels "overwhelmed" by the
   amount of work she has to do. She notes on occasion
   her heart beating "so fast" that she has to take a break
   from what she is doing. She feels her anxiety is starting
   to get in the way of her productivity. On exam, she is
   visibly anxious. A fine tremor is noted. Blood pressure is
   128/72, respirations are 16, pulse 95, and temperature
   98.6 °F. What is the next best step in management?
   A. Order TSH
   B. Prescribe lorazepam and advise to take as needed
   C. Refer to psychiatry
   D. Reassure her that once she adjusts to the new
      position she will start to feel better

3. A 52-year-old man with type II diabetes mellitus and hypertension comes in for his annual physical. He denies any acute complaints other than mild nausea. His current medications include glyburide and lisinopril. On exam, blood pressure is 138/85, respirations are 15, pulse is 90, and temperature is 97.5 °F. BUN is 30. Creatinine is 2.2. Calcium is 8. Parathyroid hormone is 95 (10–65 pg/mL). What is the most likely cause of this patient's lab abnormalities?

A. CKD
B. Primary hyperparathyroidism
C. Granulomatous disease
D. Drug-induced

Notes

ANSWERS: What Would Gunner Jess/Jim Do?

1. WWGJD? A 45-year-old man comes in for a routine health exam. He was last seen 3 years ago, when he was diagnosed with hyperlipidemia. He was placed on atorvastatin, but admits not being compliant with his cholesterol medication. He notes **increased urinary frequency, most notably at night.** He denies changes in his vision or chest pain. However, he has recently noticed his **feet have been "feeling funny."** The patient is a truck driver and mainly eats on the road. On physical exam, his blood pressure is 132/84, respiration is 16, pulse is 95, and temperature is 98.7 °F. **BMI 32.** Distal pulses are intact. **A monofilament test showed decreased sensation in his right toes.** What is the most likely cause of this patient's complaints?

Answer: B.

Explanation: An obese man with a complaint of increased urinary frequency, especially at night, and signs of peripheral neuropathy likely has diabetes mellitus.

    A. Urinary incontinence → Incorrect. Overactive bladder could increase urinary frequency. However, a monofilament test would be normal. In addition, people with overactive bladder tend to feel the urge to urinate at any time of the day.

    C. Peripheral vascular disease → Incorrect. Vascular disease could cause neuropathy. However, this patient's distal pulses were intact.

    D. Psychogenic polydipsia → Incorrect. Excessive water intake could increase urinary frequency. However, you would not expect an abnormal monofilament test.

2. WWGJD? A 38-year-old administrative assistant comes into the office with a complaint of increasing **anxiety.** She states she was recently promoted to administrative assistant in a law firm and, as a result, has taken on much more responsibility. At times she feels "overwhelmed" by the amount of work she has to do. She notes on occasion her **heart beating "so fast"** that she has to take a break from what she is doing. She feels her anxiety is starting to get in the way of her productivity. On exam, she is **visibly anxious. A fine tremor** is noted. Blood pressure is 128/72, respirations are 16, pulse 95, and temperature 97.6 °F. What is the next best step in management?

Answer: A.

    Explanation: Hyperthyroidism is more common in women than men. Common symptoms include anxiety, palpitations, and tremor. TSH is the most sensitive test to determine thyroid function.

    B. Prescribe lorazepam and advise to take as needed → Incorrect. Short-acting benzodiazepines are associated with an increased risk of dependence. Though this patient could have an underlying issue of anxiety, the next best step would be to look for a metabolic cause. In addition, selective serotonin reuptake inhibitors tend to be the gold standard for anxiety treatment.

    C. Refer to psychiatry → Incorrect. Referring to psychiatry is not necessary at this time. Based on the patient's symptoms, the next best step would be to check for a metabolic cause.

    D. Reassure her that once she adjusts to the new position she will start to feel better → Incorrect. Reassurance is not appropriate given the patient's symptoms.

3. WWGJD? A 52-year-old man with type II diabetes mellitus and hypertension comes in for his annual physical. He denies any acute complaints other than mild nausea. His current medications include glyburide and lisinopril. On exam, blood pressure is 138/85, respirations are 15, pulse is 90, and temperature is 97.5 °F. BUN is 30. Creatinine is 2.2. Calcium is 8. Parathyroid hormone is 95 (10–65 pg/mL). What is the most likely cause of this patient's lab abnormalities?

Answer: A.

    Explanation: CKD is the most common cause of secondary hyperparathyroidism. This patient's creatinine is 2.2 and he has the two most significant risk factors for CKD (diabetes and hypertension).

    B. Primary hyperparathyroidism → Incorrect. Calcium would be high, not low, in an individual with primary hyperparathyroidism.

    C. Granulomatous disease → Incorrect. In granulomatous diseases (e.g., sarcoidosis), parathyroid hormone would be low and calcium would be high.

    D. Drug-induced → Incorrect. ACE inhibitors can cause hypocalcemia. However, it tends to be more mild. And, given the patient's elevated creatinine, it's more likely that his CKD is the cause of the hyperparathyroidism.

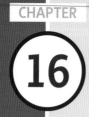

Gunner Jim's Guide to Exam Day Success

Hao-Hua Wu and Leo Wang

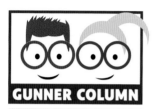

Do these three things to perform well on any shelf:

1. Master one review book
2. Do as many quality questions as you can
3. Excel like a Gunner

"Master One Review Book"

The Family Medicine shelf is known to be one of the most comprehensive exams that spans pediatrics, medicine, and ob/gyn. For this reason, students find this test to be one of the most difficult to study for. One of the most important things to do here, to get this breadth, is to find a good review book and stick to it. Remember to focus on diseases that get managed in outpatient settings, and on prophylactic and screening measurements.

Most of your learning occurs when you complete questions, so do not be discouraged if you cannot memorize every word of your review book like you did for step 1—this is not possible, even for the most accomplished physicians. Instead, use your review book as a point of reference and annotate the margins.

If you see one topic come up on multiple chapters (or maybe even multiple shelf exams), make sure to write down the page numbers where it appears, and flip to those pages every time you review. The more connections you make, the more you will master.

In addition, highlight themes that keep coming up. Any time patients in the question stem have recently changed their medication regimen, suspect the medication change as the cause of their symptoms until proven otherwise. These organizing principles transcend individual topics and can help you do well on any shelf exam test question.

"Do As Many Quality Questions As You Can"

The key to success is practicing in an environment that simulates the pressure of test day. And nothing simulates that pressure better than taking practice questions under stringent time constraints.

After you identify your review book, select as many authoritative question banks as you can. We recommend Gunner Practice, UWorld, and NBME Clinical Science practice exams. Do at least 10 questions per day under timed conditions (1.5 minutes per question) starting on the first day of your rotation.

Remember, you can complete the same question multiple times in the course of study! In fact, it is recommended that you retry the questions you got wrong in the first place, just so you know you would get it right on the test.

It is also important that the questions you complete are of high quality. This means that the length and content of the question stems reflect what you would actually see on test day. Many question bank resources are too easy (giving you a false sense of confidence) or ask about material that would not show up on the exam (wasting your time).

Once you have selected your question bank resources, count the total number of questions and divide it by the number of days you have available to study. Then make sure you set a study plan where you can make at least two passes through your questions. The first pass is completion of all available questions. The second pass is completion of all the questions you got wrong or made a lucky guess at during your first pass. Seeing how many of the second-pass questions you get correct should be a nice confidence boost leading into exam day.

As you do the questions, jot down patterns associated with the chief complaint. NBME question writers are instructed to write questions with a chief complaint that can be plausibly associated with at least five different diseases. Sharpen your differential after you read a question's first sentence and then use Buzz Words to narrow down your diagnosis. Once you reach your diagnosis, you will either be done with the question or have to draw upon knowledge of PPx, MoD, Dx, and Tx/Mgmt.

"Excel Like a Gunner"

How you take notes for the questions you complete is imperative to success.

The most effective strategy is to pick **one** take-home point for every question you complete and record it on an Excel sheet specific for your clinical rotation.

For instance, if you answer a question wrong about the treatment of bacterial vaginosis, write "Tx of bacterial vaginosis" in column A of your Excel sheet and then "metronidazole" in column B of your Excel sheet. This allows you to create an immediate, pseudo flashcard. When you review this material the following week, you can put your cursor over column A, say the answer out loud, and check your answer by shifting your cursor to column B. This saves time and emphasizes the most important takeaway for each question. You can also make your own flash cards on the Gunner Goggles iOS app.

If you understand everything in the question and answer choices, don't record it in the Excel sheet.

If you do not understand multiple things in the question and answer choices, record the most important takeaway point and move on. For test day, it is better to be confident in what you know well than to undermine your confidence by fixating on what you are weak at.

By test day, you should have one Excel sheet that contains one important take-home point from every question you were unsure about. The tabs on the bottom should be organized by question bank resource. This Excel sheet would ideally only take 3–4 hours to review, and is something you would go over the day before the exam.

Last, but not least, **trust the process.** Students often enter test day anxious and overwhelmed, which can cause them to second-guess their answer choices. Trust the process—trust that you will have covered everything leading up to the shelf exam, and have some faith in your answer selections; for these reasons, don't second-guess yourself. Your first instinct is usually right.

In summary: Read, Apply, and Review. And prepare for success on test day!

Index

Note: Page numbers followed by "f" indicate figures, "t" indicate tables, "b" indicate boxes.